HOME
BIRTHS

Published by Lonely Scribe
www.lonelyscribe.co.uk

First published 2006

Cover design and typesetting
copyright © 2006 Armadillo Design Ltd

ISBN-10:   1-905179-02-2
ISBN-13:   978-1-905179-02-2

HOME BIRTHS

stories to inspire and inform

Edited by Abigail Cairns

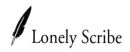 Lonely Scribe

To Mum

For starting it all

Contents

Acknowledgements

I would like to give my sincere thanks to everyone who contributed to this book for their generosity in sharing their experiences, and their enthusiasm in helping this project become a reality.

My thanks go, in particular, to my husband, Tom, who has provided countless hours of help along with his expertise in design and publishing.: for being a wonderful partner in life, an inspiring father and for making our experience of birth everything I wanted it to be. This book truly would not exist were it not for his support and enthusiasm for my ideas and his commitment to helping me achieve all my goals.

Introduction

Childbirth is one of the most miraculous and life-changing events we face. It is an experience that transcends the everyday and elicits some of our most primal responses. It has the power to redefine our very sense of self.

This book was conceived out of both a professional and a very personal interest in natural, active birth. On a professional level, as a student midwife, I felt that the book would be a valuable resource for women and their partners both in making their birthing choices and in communicating their wishes to those around them. On a personal level, it gave me the opportunity to express the wonder of natural birth at home, and share with a much wider audience the amazingly powerful effect of reading positive, affirming birth stories.

I was inspired in part by a speech I heard at a conference hosted by the Royal College of Midwives. Dame Karlene Davis, the General Secretary of the RCM, told us that as students we should 'be political', engage with the issues surrounding our chosen profession and stand up for those beliefs that we feel to be at the heart of maternity care. Insofar as I have chosen to create a work focusing on choice, and in particular on the minority who choose a home birth, this book could be said to be a political statement. I certainly hope that I am fulfilling her request by promoting home birth as a real choice for parents, even though, as some of these stories show, the decision is not always supported by the health professionals involved.

Grantly Dick Read, in his *Revelation of Childbirth*, was one of the first authors to declare his belief in empowering and improving women's birthing experiences through education and information, hence ceding control of birth to women. It is in this spirit that I produce this wonderful collection of moving and intimate stories of real home birth experiences.

On a personal level, my twin sister and I fell pregnant only two months apart and so spent most of our pregnancies together. We discovered an insatiable appetite for everything and anything connected to pregnancy and birth, and in particular birth stories. We simply couldn't get enough. Yet when we began to think of planning our births at home, we found very few actual stories to give us an emotional insight into what we could hope to expect.

Like many of the contributors to this book, we came across a number of dedicated proponents of natural birth who fired our enthusiasm all the more (see the list of suggested further reading at the back of this book). With some research online we found discussions on how to plan a home birth, and various academic descriptions of risk and benefits. But it quickly became clear that there is a relative lack of direct narrative that speaks to pregnant women and their partners on an emotional level. In today's culture hospital birth has become the standard for normality, so inevitably the information available to expectant parents is largely based on this experience of birth. What we craved were real, in-depth descriptions of what women and their partners experienced in the home environment.

I discovered what became my bible in pregnancy when I came across a dusty, crumbling edition of Ina May Gaskin's *Spiritual Midwifery* on the shelf in my mentor's office while out working on a placement in the community. Reading it, I was swept away into a world of colourful, powerful, sensual, even sexual descriptions of the wonders of natural childbirth. It struck a chord in me that has been humming ever since: this is the way it can be; this is what women like me want, and indeed what some lucky women even manage to achieve in this modern world of technological birth. I wanted to tell the whole world about it, and so I set about doing just that, in whatever small way I could.

* * *

The stories in this book have come from a variety of geographical locations around the UK (and one from far-flung New Zealand), and as such reflect a range of different viewpoints. Clearly only those who chose to share their experiences are represented, and as such this not a true cross-section of all of those who choose home birth. However, it was specifically not my intention to produce an academic work, rather to share with a wider audience the joy and wonder of birth at home.

The contributors describe their experiences in the context of the much wider social group to which expectant parents inevitably belong, incorporating a whole host of characters from friends, family and work colleagues to a range of health professionals. The term *psycho-social support* is wordy, but describes the need we all have to belong to and make use of the network of social relationships which surrounds us in our daily lives. Our social context has a huge impact on the choices we make, and these stories demonstrate the broad range of attitudes that people choosing home birth can encounter, from sceptical and negative to supportive and encouraging.

Several of the stories draw attention to the commonly expressed assumption that birth at home is inherently risky. Many authors were offended by explicit and implicit suggestions that they were being irresponsible, and that by choosing a home birth they were putting their babies' lives at risk for the sake of their own preferences or aspirations. These stories demonstrate that, in fact, those who choose home births tend to be very aware of current research and are usually highly informed about the risks and benefits of their decision not to use medical facilities.

It was important for me to provide a realistic image of home birth, so as not to be accused of idealism (God forbid!), and there are a number of stories that depict planned home births where women subsequently transferred into hospital for a variety of medical reasons. Indeed, most of the contributors take pains to reassure the reader that, contrary to the image of reckless risk-taking, they are fully prepared to acknowledge if they need extra medical attention and would heed their midwife's expert opinion and transfer to hospital if the situation called for it.

In looking at this decision-making process, as with other aspects of home birth, I felt it was important to include a section on partners' perspectives. This is an area that is often overlooked, though I have found that partners enjoy talking about their birth experiences just as much as the mothers do. By including their side of the story I hope to address some of the particular concerns that partners reading this book may have about home birth.

What comes across in this section is the way in which home is often a much more inclusive environment than hospital for those with the dual role of partner and parent. It interests me that even though some partners describe feeling the lack of an active role in labour, they are evidently much more at ease in their own surroundings. They can engage in other activities to make them feel useful and involved (providing essential refreshments to the midwives, usually!). The photo essay is of particular interest, since I am told that it wasn't always possible to take birth pictures in hospital at that time. These beautiful images might never have existed were it not for the fact that the parents chose a home birth.

I have chosen to include some stories from the 1960s and 1970s alongside more contemporary accounts in order to show how medical attitudes towards birth are constantly evolving. Although some of the attitudes and practices described are no longer prevalent, they show the constantly shifting face of maternity care and highlight the variety of choices that women are able to make these days.

One of the more practical considerations of home birth is the decision parents make about extended family being present. Several stories describe the choices families made as to whether or not they wanted their other children present during their labours and births, and also the choices children themselves made when asked their preference. In many cases, but significantly not all, the parents chose not to have their children present. Some explain that they simply didn't want the distraction of having to focus on someone else's needs at this crucial time; others share their anxiety that their labour might frighten their young children. However, more often than not, children are included in some part of the labouring process or are present very soon after the birth, and in every case this is seen as one of the great rewards of home birth. The opportunity for our children to witness and understand childbirth in a positive, empowering light, is surely a worthy ambition.

Some of the contributors to the book were themselves born at home; others describe how hearing the birth narratives of friends or relatives helped in forming their own opinions. These anecdotal references demonstrate the effect of positive story telling in action, which was one of the prime motivators in bringing together this collection for publication. The tendency of the media is to make drama out of significant life events such as birth and death, often by focusing on their negative aspects. Calm, even blissful, birth is relatively under-represented, which

I believe seriously undermines parents' expectations of their birthing abilities.

It has been heartwarming to discover how many women not only share my passion for natural home birth, but are willing to share their deeply personal experiences for the benefit of others facing this life-changing event. One contributor summed up her motivation in the letter that arrived with her stories:

> *I hope this book will help to change the attitudes of the vast majority who are too scared or view home birth as irresponsible to see that we are a very aware group of people who make the decision to birth where we feel safest and happiest… If my four very different births offer comfort or affirmation to just one woman who then goes on to deliver at home and passes that joy on by telling her story to others then I will feel I've made a real difference.*

I

Women's Voices

Hannah F's story

Rohan, 2005

At 1:30 in the morning I woke up with powerful sensations in my lower abdomen… Somewhere inside I knew this was it, but I held back my excitement and waited. After half an hour I woke my husband, Ameet, knowing that he would be my rock throughout what was to come.

"I think I'm having contractions," I said. Ameet woke himself up. The pain was strong but manageable and we swung into action. Ameet got a watch, and we timed the contractions which were roughly four minutes apart and lasting thirty seconds. They were quite regular. I felt a bit apologetic about calling the midwives at this hour, but of course this wasn't the time to be polite. We know of two women who had thirty-minute labours!

Our first midwife, Vanda, arrived at 3:00. Now the sensations, which I can't describe (tightening, pain, overpowering) were more frequently spaced. Ameet and I had started chanting 'Maaaaaaaa' together with each one. We were to keep this up for the next seven and a half hours! I breathed in deeply and the exhalation was as long as could be, while the sound kept me grounded, safe and relaxed.

Ameet sometimes held me close to him, more so as the labour progressed, and the sound he made as he chanted maaaaaa was lovely and deep and comforting. The best pain relief ever. Maaaaa maaaa maaaa. 'Ma' is the word for mother in so many languages, including the yogic language of Sanskrit, and so for us, as yoga teachers, it felt right.

I don't know what Vanda made of us! She examined me once between contractions and I was 3cm dilated. Then she left us alone for a couple more hours, assuring us she was only ten minutes away. I was a little nervous as I was clear my labour was in full swing now, but also I had real faith that this birth would be fine.

I spent some time in the bath. The warm water was wonderful. When a contraction came I called to Ameet, who was preparing the sitting room for the main event, and we chanted together. Time was very vague, marked only by the space from one opening of my cervix to the next. I was in my own inner space, mentally focused and bearing the pain of the contractions.

Ameet laid out yoga mats, an exercise ball, towels and cushions in our labour room, and dimmed the lights. He prepared the TENS machine for me. I got out of the bath at some point, and Vanda returned at some other point – I can't remember the order! She suggested another internal exam and I agreed – curious – as the first hadn't been uncomfortable. I was full of anticipation as she moved her fingers over my cervix, hoping to God that all the pain hadn't been in vain. When Vanda said I was 8cm dilated I was elated. Things were going really well. I was still relaxed and positive.

By now I was in the sitting room, TENS machine turned on, standing and rotating my hips as I had done for so many months in my yoga practice. Sometimes I sat and rocked on the exercise ball, and sometimes I knelt down. Ameet was helping me by being close and calm, and supporting me physically when I wanted him to. I heard the neighbours getting up and leaving their homes for work. What do they think of us, chanting so loudly? I wondered. I didn't mind one bit.

Then, just as I began to think the pain was changing to the urge to push, Vanda left us and three new women walked in. Two were midwives and one was a student nurse, but I didn't take this in at the time. I felt disrupted by their presence. They were full of the morning energy, bright and sociable, and I was somewhere in the out-there space of transition. As it happened they were lovely, but it took me a while to fully trust in the new dynamic.

Now my labour became more difficult. I began to think, how can I possibly be about to give birth to a baby? I felt totally unprepared for this! It just felt impossible that I could push a baby out of me. I got mentally stuck. Instead of chanting, now I started yelling. Jo, one of the midwives, urged me to keep my sounds low and direct the energy downwards "like you're doing a poo". I felt a bit lost, as the urge to bear down wasn't very clear to me. I went to the toilet on my own and felt a massive urge to push then. "Don't have the baby down the loo!" Jo called. I came back to the living room.

It took over two hours of pushing. I was hanging on to Ameet for what felt like dear life. I remember thinking, this might kill me, I might just die with the effort. I was really exhausted. As time went on and my contractions got weaker and more spaced apart I could sense that the midwives were getting concerned. Would I be able to deliver this baby without hospital and intervention?

Then our baby's head crowned. "I can see the hair!" Jo said. Ameet was amazed. "The baby's got black hair!" he gasped. It was such an exciting and rewarding moment. The pushing was working! I put my hand down and touched my baby's head. It was amazing to feel the round wetness of this precious little head. Then Jo realised that we were touching the membrane, and that my waters still hadn't broken. Ameet and I tore gently at the membrane and some water trickled out.

I kept pushing and pushing. I was kneeling and leaning against the sofa when Jo suggested I turn around. This seemed impossible, but I did it and now, on all fours, I pushed again with all my might. Ameet was praying silently for this to be it. Suddenly, without me being aware of pushing, I felt myself split and my baby's head was free. Everybody was exclaiming, "The baby's here." And then with a delicious schloooping feeling *he* was born!

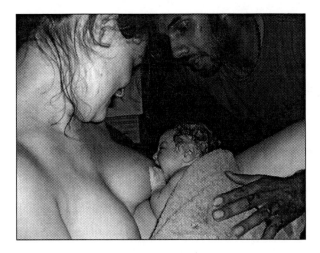

Ameet passed him through my legs and my life changed as I saw him for the first time. I couldn't believe how beautiful he looked, and how strong and healthy he was. He was gorgeous. I sat against the sofa and held my baby. I couldn't take my eyes off him. He nuzzled at my nipple and we took each other in softly, skin to skin. What magic!

After half an hour Ameet took him and I lifted myself up for my placenta to come out. Plop! Easy.

"We're trying out the name Rohan," we agreed, and so Rohan came into our lives.

For another perspective on this experience, you can read Ameet's story on p.257

Ann's story

Reisha, 2000

In May 1999 I discovered that I was pregnant; I had been reacting to normally pleasant smells in a strange way for a few weeks but had no idea that I was actually pregnant. My partner and I had been together for less than a year so becoming a family was not something we had actively discussed.

My original birth plan had included a hospital birth. Even though my partner, Reggie, had been born at home, and so had most of his siblings, we did not really consider my having a home birth. I thought every woman gave birth in hospital and my midwife had not openly discussed other options. My twin sister was pregnant at the same time – 20 weeks ahead of me – and she too was giving birth in hospital.

The turning point for my decision to have a home birth came when my sister gave birth. I visited her in hospital a few hours after her daughter was born and at this point I really changed my mind about a hospital birth. I found the atmosphere to be very sterile, there was no real bonding with a particular midwife and the whole natural experience of childbirth felt so clinical and medical.

By the time I had my next antenatal appointment I had totally changed my birth plan: I wanted a home birth and had already looked at the option of water birth. Reggie was very supportive of this: we were both (and still are) very much in favour of as little intervention as possible and both believe in complementary medicine and practices. I feel these beliefs wouldn't have been respected in hospital and I might have ended up having intervention during the delivery.

My midwife left the GP's practice and the newly appointed midwife was very supportive of a home birth. The GP I saw, however, was not. She was not in favour of home births, nor was the consultant I saw at the City Hospital. He did his best to persuade me to change my mind and opt for a hospital birth. One of his main arguments was that he felt my cervix would not dilate fully and this would complicate a home delivery.

The lack of support I got for my option of a home birth was not very helpful – I felt like I was not allowed to make a choice and it made me feel inadequate. If I had not wanted a home birth so strongly, I think I would have been persuaded to go to hospital. But I can be a very stubborn person and was definitely not changing my mind – I preferred to let nature take its course.

As far as I can remember my family supported my decision but did wonder why I wasn't going into hospital. The fact that I lived about a mile down the road from the City Hospital put their minds more at rest. I, however, wasn't going to change my mind unless complications arose during the birth, then of course I would have gone into hospital.

My pregnancy went extremely well after I had got over my period of morning sickness. I had developed a nice little bump and did not suffer from any stretch marks and only had one day of swollen ankles. I was training as an aromatherapist at the time and used my oils to benefit my body during pregnancy. I also saw a homoeopath during pregnancy and had remedies prescribed for after the birth. Our birthing pool had been hired about a month before the birth and was just awaiting assembly in our kitchen.

The only slightly worrying factor for me as my labour became imminent, and more so since baby was overdue, was the fact that the hospital had given me a date to be induced and my midwife was away on holiday. I was a bit anxious because it meant I did not know which midwives would be present at the birth. I definitely did not want to be induced and thankfully my labour pains started just in time.

By the evening of Sunday 23 January, my contractions were getting much closer together so I telephoned the number I had been given for the midwife on duty that night. I did not know at that time that I would bond with her so well, but when I spoke to her I knew instantly that she would be really supportive of home births. As soon as she arrived at our home I really liked her – she was so relaxed and helpful.

The birth pool was slowly filling with water, ready for me to get in. I had tremendous pains around my spinal column – when the midwife checked me out she said that our baby was nose to spine, hence the searing pains I was feeling. She suggested I get into the pool, and I felt more relaxed in the water. The pain was not taken away – somehow I thought it would have been – but when I was checked again a bit later on, our baby had turned and was now facing the right way.

Up to this point I had been breathing in essential oils to help with the pain relief and nothing else: I reacted very badly to gas and air and couldn't use this option. So no feeling high for me! Being in water felt more secure than kneeling on my living room carpet. The sensation of the warm water around me made me more relaxed and it definitely had a positive effect on our baby – the baby's stress levels were monitored and there was no stress so someone was definitely happy.

I sat down in the pool for a while, and then changed positions to kneeling. At this point a second midwife arrived. I had met her once before at a clinic. The midwives worked well together and obviously knew each other. They both helped me with my breathing and were very encouraging.

During the whole labour period Reggie was very supportive. He massaged me and was very encouraging in the way he spoke to me. I was in a lot of pain, especially during the final labour stage. I remember I had real urges to push too much and found it very difficult not to. Nobody had told me that I would hurt so much – I felt as if I had been cut open and salt had been rubbed into my wounds. This sensation lasted for what seemed an eternity. I kept wanting to push too early – I just wanted the sensation to go away.

This last stage of labour really dragged on, but when it was finally time for me to push nothing would stop me and at 5:20am on Monday 24 January 2000, our baby was finally born. I remember crying a lot at this stage. I had given birth sitting on the bottom of the pool with my legs apart. The final stages of the birth were recorded on video. Baby, who was called Reisha, had finally arrived and was absolutely perfect.

I stayed in the pool for a while because I had decided to deliver the placenta naturally as well. This happened only 13 minutes after Reisha arrived, and I delivered it on the mats around the pool. I can vividly remember the large amount of blood on my kitchen floor.

Both midwives were fantastic throughout – I don't think I could have done so well without their support. They had both had experience of water births in hospital and home births, but neither had done a home water birth (a first time for everything!). They both praised me for having an intervention-free birth and said that more women should opt for home births.

I feel that by having a home birth, I was able to bond much more quickly with my baby. She was not taken away from me to be cleaned and because I was in my own surroundings she was not subjected to any stress. Plus, her daddy was present throughout the whole experience, which was great for him and for me as well. I loved the fact that I only had to go upstairs to my own bed afterwards, and that people could visit whenever they wanted without any restrictions. And Reisha was not subjected to the sterile smells and sounds that are always present in hospitals.

I have absolutely no regrets about having chosen a home birth. In fact I feel very lucky to have been able to fulfil my birth plan: I had chosen a home water birth, with no pain relief, and had no interventions and no complications afterwards. I don't think that many women are as lucky as I was. I feel that God was smiling on me the day I gave birth.

The only real thing that I would have changed in hindsight is that, when Reisha was born into the water, I would have preferred it if she had been allowed to stay underwater for longer before being brought up to breathe. I would have found this more natural. Still, this one little thing does not detract from perhaps the most special thing I have ever done in my whole life. I feel very proud that I went through so much pain and still allowed my body to feel everything.

Home births should be encouraged far more than they are. What better place to give birth than in one's own surroundings? Hospitals are great if there are any complications, but otherwise nature does its job and there really is no need for all this medical intervention.

Corinne's story

Oliver, 1979

I knew as soon as I woke up that I was in labour. It was about 6:00am, but you get used to getting up at that time with three children to get ready for school. The contractions were already well established so we swung into action straight away. We thought it might be quite quick because the twins, born four years before, had arrived with unseemly haste in only three hours.

At last I was going to get the home birth I had always wanted. I had tried for one with the first, but the medical profession thirty years ago was deeply unhappy about first births at home, so I had caved in to the pressure and agreed to a hospital birth. It had been fine, but not home. And of course thirty years ago a hospital birth meant being shaved, given an enema, a virtually routine episiotomy, and an injection in the upper thigh which you hardly noticed to help with the afterbirth. So I got the full set.

Second time around I booked for a home birth. And everything was going swimmingly with the pregnancy until twins were suddenly found at 36 weeks! The home birth went out of the window. Luckily this was a very quick birth and I was nearly fully dilated by the time I got to the hospital so I managed to miss out on the shaving, etc, etc. And with two healthy seven-pound babies I could have managed perfectly well at home. But I did understand that with twins there is a lot more that can go wrong. The only thing I really did not understand was the necessity for these two hulking great full-term babies to go into the Special

Care Unit, simply because it was routine for twins. I kicked up a stink and got them released about twelve hours later. They could have been there for 48 hours!

So this time I was finally going to get the chance to do it my way. We got the children dressed and ready for school, and rang friends to arrange for after-school care.

The bedroom was ideal: large enough to wander about, and with an en-suite bathroom. It was on the third floor at the back of the house, so no road or other outside noise, and with a lovely dormer window for looking at the blue sky. And it was a lovely sunny day.

We had the Mozart ready on the cassette player on the windowsill, in case I needed calming or inspiration. When I was later asked if I wanted any music I just shook my head: I wanted to concentrate.

The midwife arrived promptly, at about 9:30am. One of the old school: calmly efficient and no nonsense. I thought she would pop in to see how I was getting on and then disappear for a few hours. But once she was there she stayed; a quite calm figure sitting in the corner watching.

I was up and about, walking up and down the room, with occasional breaks on the bed for checks. All was fine. I really worked hard at all the relaxation, concentration, and breathing I had learnt (and taught) at NCT lessons. I had been an NCT teacher for several years and was a strong advocate of the natural way of childbirth.

And all continued to be fine hour in, hour out. So no quick labour then! Eventually, at about midday I began to feel really uncomfortable and took to the bed, lying on my right side, propped up on lots of pillows and grateful for the gas and air. By 1:00 I was fully-dilated and ready to push… and push… and push… and push.

My baby's head was facing the front, and I had a long painful wait while he turned all the way round. By the end I was shouting at the midwife, "This bloody baby is never going to come out!" But as soon as he had turned his head was ready to crown. The midwife told me to put my hand down to feel the head. I was stunned. I could actually feel my baby before he was born. Two more pushes and the head was out. The shoulders took a bit of work before the rest of my new baby boy (oh, how I had wanted a boy!) was out. It was 3:15pm and I had a 9lb 15oz baby, with a huge head and a face so squashed that he was unable to open his eyes for about three days.

The midwife finished off, but was unsure whether I would need stitches for the small tear, so I had to wait for a doctor to come out. Apparently only men knew how to do the sewing!

There is a very special feeling to lying back in your own bed with your new baby. It all feels totally right. And not long afterwards the girls came back. Five-year-old Miranda first, with a look on her face which is almost indescribable in its utter joy. Then the four-year-old twins Abigail and Verity, not so overwhelmed, but full of self-importance at having a new brother. And Chris, my husband, had a wonderful set of photographs of the whole thing for us to look back on. What a way to complete the family!

For another perspective on this experience, you can see Chris's photo-essay on p.262

Tracy's stories

Max, 2002

I had two children aged ten and twelve from a previous marriage, who were both born in hospital. When I found out I was expecting again I was very keen to see if I could have a home birth. I would have liked one with my second child but was told that it wasn't supported by the doctors or midwives at the time. That was back in 1991.

So I was really delighted when I visited my midwife to hear that she totally supported home births. In order for me to have one I would have to fit certain medical criteria for my own and the baby's safety. These included: that labour did not start earlier than two weeks before the due date or later than two weeks after the due date; that my blood pressure was not a problem; and that there were no other problems, such as breech presentation.

The main reason I wanted a home birth was that both my previous labours had been quick and uncomplicated: the first one lasting six hours, the second only two. My second labour was extremely intense and I remember finding it very difficult being in the car on the way to hospital then having to get out and into the labour suite as my contractions came thick and fast without any apparent break between them.

I talked with Paul about it and I think he was a little worried about whether everything would be all right and what would happen if something went wrong. I also talked with a neighbour who had recently delivered her second child at home and she said it was a lovely experience. My friends and family, however, thought I was mad.

We discussed the issue with our community midwife, Elaine, who was very reassuring. She told us if there were any concerns or problems we could always change our minds at the last minute and go to hospital.

My labour started following a hot bath. My waters broke and I called Paul straight away. I was worried that he wouldn't get home quickly enough and that the labour would progress very quickly. His sister came to fetch the older two children as they didn't want to be present and we were happy about that.

The midwife on duty was called Jackie and she came out to visit. My first impression of her was that she was a lovely lady. She checked me over and said I was 3cm dilated although there were no apparent contractions. So it was to be a waiting game. She went home and phoned the second midwife to advise her that it looked like it would be an early morning call.

We sat on the settee waiting for what seemed like hours, although it was in fact only half an hour later that the contractions started, and Paul phoned straightaway for Jackie's return. The contractions were coming very quickly. I remember getting quite distressed because it seemed like ages before Jackie arrived although it was probably only 20 minutes or so from when we called. The pain was running away with me. Jackie came straight in and put her hand on my back and said, "It's okay Tracy, I'm here now." They were the most comforting words anyone could have said to me at that time and I felt my whole body relax for just a second before the next contraction started.

She checked me over and then I felt I wanted to push so off we went. At some point Maria, the second midwife, arrived and she monitored the baby's heartbeat between the contractions. I was kneeling over the dining room chair on the floor of the living room. An hour and 15 minutes later Max was born.

I wanted Max to be given to me between my legs but it was strategically quite difficult. Jackie told me not to sit back but I instinctively did. My legs were really shaking and poor little Max was nearly squashed. He lay quite still in front of me and I remember panicking because I didn't think he was breathing. I asked Jackie if he was alright and she said he was fine, he just needed a minute: he was breathing and was just coming to after his rapid birth. Again, seconds seemed like minutes and then he started to cry. I sat back and cuddled him. We were both naked. Labour gets me very hot! The cord was cut and he was passed over to Maria who checked him out while Jackie delivered the placenta and checked me over. All was fine: thankfully no stitches!

I put Max to the breast and he nuzzled in straight away. It was then time to get him dressed as we didn't want him to get cold. Maria did that for us. I was a bit nervous as it had been a long time since I had dressed a newborn. The midwives cleared all the mess up and took everything away and then sat and had a nice cup of tea and a chat with us. It was just so lovely and homely. I enjoyed my time in hospital with the first two but they were in a bland room on a hospital bed with midwives and doctors popping in every so often. This time it was just us and it was lovely. We found out that this was Jackie's first home delivery and that she and I shared the same birthday! What a coincidence: it seems that it was meant to be.

Jackie was a lovely calm midwife to have had with us. I was really scared at the speed the contractions were coming, and there was absolutely no way I could have got into a car and gone to hospital. I was very fortunate to have had such a quick and totally textbook labour. The only thing I wished had happened was the gas and air. I didn't get any. It would have made the pain just that bit bearable, but in fairness to Jackie she was straight into it from the moment she arrived. She could hear I was beginning to get distressed, the contractions were no more than a minute apart and relentless. The gas cylinders had only made it just inside the front door.

About an hour after the birth Maria left and after about two hours Jackie left. We were on our own with our little baby. Wow! If we had been in hospital Paul would have had to leave me at the ward door since it was night time. It was so nice that we could just be together without interruptions in our own rooms, drinking our own tea, and I felt quite elated at what had just happened. When Jackie told us to go to bed and sleep we thought she was mad. How could we go to sleep? We'd just had a baby. We lay for a long time in bed just watching him.

Martha, 2005

When we found out we were expecting again there was no question of us having anything other than a home birth. I was a bit shaken after Max's birth as the labour was more intense that I remembered which made me quite nervous going into labour with Martha, but on reflection hers was the nicest one. Elaine was still our community midwife and all through the pregnancy she was determined that she would deliver our baby! A lovely thought, but would we be lucky enough to reach D-Day when she was on duty?

At around seven months I had a possible problem with my a suspected pulmonary oedema which put me in hospital for a few days while they checked things out. I struck up a lovely relationship with the midwives, one in particular whose name was Marian. The hospital had changed and the maternity ward was now a purpose-built unit, much nicer than the older part of the hospital I had delivered my first two children in. As the test results turned out to be negative there was no problem with me delivering at home again.

One afternoon I felt a trickle of water. No contractions though. I was very nervous this time because of the speed of Max's birth: I was really anxious not be on my own and I wanted to make sure I got the gas and air. We called the midwife straight away. It wasn't Elaine. A midwife came out to check me over and said that I had had a hindwater tear. As the hours ticked by, nothing happened. I paced up and down the kitchen floor and sat on the birth ball and bounced on it trying to get things started.

The following day Elaine was on duty and she came to see me. It was just a waiting game. She had to take a swab because once there has been a break in the sack they have to ensure that there is no infection as this could harm the baby. She said that the hospital would let me go no more than 72 hours. If labour hadn't started naturally by then I would have to go in and be induced. I felt quite deflated and again didn't want to be induced, but nothing was happening.

I called Jill, my homeopath, and she came round with some remedies for me which I took while Elaine was there. All day we waited and still nothing happened. Elaine was on call that night so if anything was to happen then she would be there for me. I remember telling her, if it happens tonight just make sure you give me the gas and air! I was most insistent. Poor Elaine, she must have been really looking forward to the delivery!

Anyhow, at about 2:20am I suddenly sat up in bed. Paul had to pull me up because my waters gushed as I had a contraction and I ran to the loo shouting to him to call Elaine as well as his sister, Jo (she was there in 5 minutes – boy, she was fast!). I jumped in the shower to ease the contractions while the older two children left. Then I went downstairs. The contractions rapidly reduced from every 5 minutes, to 4, 3, 2, 1. Paul's face was a picture. I remember looking at him and thinking 'He thinks he going to be delivering this baby at this rate!'

Elaine arrived around 3am. She lives a fair distance away and the car was iced up. I immediately bellowed, "Gas and air, give me the gas and air!" She was rushing like mad as the contractions were obviously very intense. I inhaled and my shoulders just relaxed and I wanted to push. Elaine said, "Go with it, you know what you're doing." She didn't get time to check me, the baby's heart beat or anything. At 3:15am Martha was born. Job done. She was wrapped in a towel and handed to Paul. The placenta was delivered and I was given the all clear. No stitches! The gas and air made a huge difference to how I felt and how I coped with the second stage of the labour.

The student midwife arrived and I put Martha to the breast. She took to it straight away. When the second midwife arrived she checked Martha over and dressed her for us. The whole event was so fast, I don't even recall her name.

It was lovely having Elaine deliver my last baby. I had built up a relationship with her while pregnant with Max and again with Martha. It was different again actually knowing the midwife who delivered our baby. She felt like a friend and the experience was very emotional and lovely to share with her. There were just the three of us. How special is that?

For another perspective on this experience, you can read Paul's story on p.233

Deborah's stories

Betty, 2003

My first birth was four years ago and although it was very straightforward, it resulted in my son being in hospital for two weeks. He was discovered to have a bowel disorder that had to be operated on at eight weeks. It had been a very traumatic time for me and I was determined that my second birth would be different.

From 20 weeks of pregnancy I planned to have a home birth, and once this decision was made I felt very excited and positive about the pending event! I primarily made the decision because of my dislike of hospitals, but also for a whole host of other reasons. I felt I would be much more relaxed at home and this would lead to an easier labour and birth. I also couldn't bear the thought of my husband having to leave the baby and me alone in the hospital – this seemed so unfair on him and not ideal for me either!

My husband realised how important this decision was to me and was behind me one hundred percent. My midwife was very supportive and seemed to be pleased that I'd be having my baby at home. She did outline a whole list of possible reasons why I might have to be transferred to hospital, but I decided to worry about these things if they occurred. She also spoke about what the midwives would 'allow' me to do, which I found a little annoying. It felt as if they were making some concession for me rather than helping me fulfil my right to the birth I chose.

Four days before my due date, I had a show and was very excited as I took this as a sign that the baby would arrive the next day (as had happened with my son). I informed my husband that he should stay home from work as the baby was coming (despite the absence of any contractions!) All night I paced up and down willing something to happen, but not a sign.

At 5am the next morning I suggested to my husband that we should do something to kick-start the labour and he rather half-heartedly tweaked my nipples. Within 30 seconds my contractions had started and they continued every three minutes!

I then began to frantically clean the house – scrubbing floors, cleaning out cupboards and generally nesting. By 7:30am we decided it was time for my son to be shipped off to a friend's house. He went willingly, although he did comment that he wasn't ready for the baby to be born that day!

We called the midwife at 8:00 and by 8:30 she had arrived with what looked like the contents of a doctors surgery. She examined me, pronounced me well on my way and summoned the help of midwife number two. By this time I was bouncing up and down on my birthing ball and beginning to feel quite uncomfortable. Midwife number two asked me if I'd like a massage and proceeded to massage my back with essential oils. It was fantastic – so relaxing and it really helped with the pain.

The midwives took a very low-key role in the proceedings. They sat and chatted to us and really put me at ease. They were both very experienced and were obviously delighted to be delivering a baby. They were also extremely encouraging and positive, telling me numerous times how well I was coping and that it wouldn't be long. At 10:30am my waters broke naturally and I moved onto the bed. I kept remembering my antenatal classes and thinking I should be in a less conventional position, but my body was telling me to lie down so that's what I did! By 10:40am I was getting the urge to push and my midwives instructed me to listen to them and do what they said. They told me they were too old to do stitches so they'd make sure I didn't tear! I completely trusted them, and when Bethan Alice was born at 10:48am I was overjoyed. She weighed a healthy 7lb 12oz (a spot on guess from midwife one), and she was beautiful.

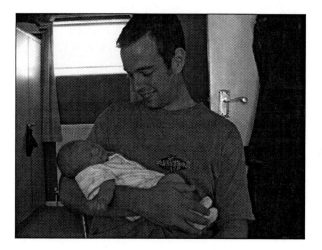

After cleaning up (although there was very little mess), running me a bath, making a cup of tea and sharing a glass of champagne, the midwives left my husband and I to enjoy our new addition. I was overwhelmed by my fantastic birth experience. I couldn't have wished for better support from the midwives and my wonderful husband. It had all felt so natural and perfect. There was no point when I felt scared as I knew I was being looked after by experienced professionals who had my best interests at heart.

The whole experience was a world away from my previous hospital birth and I would recommend it to anyone. As we sat there in bed with our hour-old baby in my arms breastfeeding happily, we knew we'd made the right decision in staying at home. When my son met his new sister, she was in our home where she belonged and I was where he'd left me. The birth was just a natural part of our everyday life and not a big trauma and upheaval.

Esther, 2005

I had never been overdue. In fact my previous two babies both arrived three days early so I was fairly confident about when number three would turn up...

At three days overdue I was slightly annoyed. At six days overdue I was thoroughly fed up! The midwife had been around and given me a sweep two days previously (not my idea of fun), and this had produced a lot of show but not much else. I was beginning to worry about the pressure to be induced and envisaged my home birth slipping away from me.

At 7:30 on Wednesday night I had my first contraction. I was shocked by how painful it was. With my previous two births the contractions had been fairly mild till the last minute but this time they were very uncomfortable from the start. I began to get excited thinking that this could be the night and debated whether or not to put the TENS machine on yet. I had about half an hour's worth of regular contractions before they died off. My very sensible husband suggested we get a good night's sleep and that maybe it would happen tomorrow, so I reluctantly went to bed. During the night I woke up three times with painful contractions but quickly went back to sleep. I got up the next morning feeling very disheartened.

Despite a few continuing contractions we decided Stuart should go to work that morning. It didn't seem like much was happening and I didn't want to be sat around waiting. I carried on with the normal routine of taking Owen to school and went for a walk with my friend Lara in an attempt to intensify the pains I was having. By lunchtime I'd got to the stage where I had a pain every time I stood up. This was frustrating as I was torn between walking around to bring it on or sitting down and resting as I was in charge of a small child.

At 2.00 my husband rang to see how I was doing. I told him I was fine and that things were much the same. Ten minutes later I rang back and asked him to come home. It wasn't because it was too painful, but I didn't feel like I'd be able to walk to school and fetch Owen without doubling over!

Stuart got home at 2:30pm and helped me put the TENS machine on before going to get Owen. We'd already arranged for the children to go to my sister's house overnight and when she picked them up at 4:30 the contractions were every five minutes. I talked to her while I was having a contraction and she told me to think positive and enjoy the gaps between contractions. This really helped me focus throughout the labour.

Things seemed to speed up from this point. I spent the time pacing around the house or leaning over the bed. I bounced on my exercise ball a bit and felt I was managing quite well. Stuart kept suggesting we ring the midwives but I felt we should hold off. At 6:00 I suddenly changed my mind and Stuart made the call.

The first midwife arrived at 6:30. Her name was Maggie and she seemed very positive and encouraging. She examined me and said I was 5-6cm dilated. She felt that the baby's arrival wasn't too far off so she rang the second midwife and told her to set off from home. The second midwife was called Hannah and it was her first night on call. She was pregnant herself and seemed very calm and unobtrusive.

The next hour or so was spent with me breathing through contractions whilst the midwives wrote notes, listened to the baby's heart rate and chatted. Maggie gave us a leaflet on 'Your emotions after childbirth', which I found very strange! She later laughed at us for actually reading it during labour. At one point they both went and sat downstairs while Stuart and I stayed in the bedroom. At this point I remember sobbing quietly whilst he cuddled me. The contractions were very intense but the breaks in between were lovely! They were still only coming every five minutes but they were getting stronger all the time. My TENS machine worked brilliantly – especially the boost button!

At about 7:45 I began to feel like the baby should soon be born. Everything hurt so much and I felt sick. It seemed like it would never be over. Maggie kept encouraging me to stand up, but every time I tried it was agony. In the end she was so insistent that I gave in. As I stood up my waters broke all over her feet! I immediately sat down again.

Once the waters had gone I began to get an urge to push. I climbed onto the bed and began pushing at 8:13pm. At this stage the contractions felt like they were tearing me apart and I had agonising pains in my sides. It was like nothing I'd ever felt before. As I pushed I grabbed hold of Stuart's hair and tugged hard – he informs me that it was very painful! Thankfully I only had to push twice before the baby's head was out, I looked down and saw a crumpled little face looking up at me! The baby had twisted at the last minute and been born facing the side instead of downwards. I was reassured to hear a loud and angry cry even before the baby was fully born. I had to push the shoulders out, which was also a new experience for me: in my previous labours they'd just slipped out.

My baby was born at 8:16pm and was delivered onto my tummy. I couldn't reach the baby because the cord was very short but once the cord was cut and the placenta delivered (aided by a Syntometrine injection) I got a cuddle.

Stuart and I gazed at the little face for a couple of minutes before the midwife said, "Do you know what you've got?" We'd forgotten to look! I hadn't noticed anything between the legs when I'd glanced down so I wasn't surprised when we discovered we'd had a beautiful little girl. We were so delighted – just what we'd wanted! We also discovered quite a big purple coloured mark on her right knee; the midwives assured us it was just a birth mark.

I put little Esther Rose to the breast straight away and she looked at me as if to say 'What do you expect me to do with that?!' She just licked it a bit before falling asleep. The midwives then weighed her and pronounced her to be 7lb 9oz.

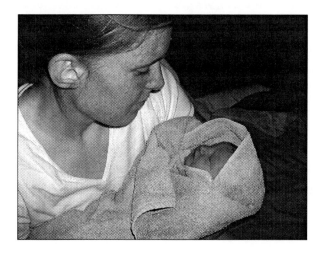

Esther had her first feed about an hour after she was born. I was amazed once more by a baby's instinct to suck and by how much I wanted to nurture and care for this little scrap of a person. When the midwives left at 9:30pm (after champagne and congratulations) Stuart and I sat and baby worshipped.

What an incredible experience! Another wonderful home birth. It was more painful than the last but just as breathtaking. I felt good: no tears, no stitches and lying peacefully in my own bed. We'd been blessed with a real beauty. A dark haired girl who looked so different to her brother and sister. We sat and gazed at her and fell in love.

Julie's story

Luisa, 2005

Initially I was planning to have my baby at a small local maternity hospital which is very close to my home. I had gone for my regular checks at this hospital up to week 25, and was discussing how we would go on when the day arrived. The idea was that I would stay at home for as long as possible and then go down there when necessary, but mostly to try and stay at home as much as possible. This started me thinking about being at home during labour and I began to realise that this was the most appealing option for me.

When I next visited the hospital I asked the midwives about the possibility of home birth and though they were very happy to go with that they mentioned there was a possibility that I would have various midwives assisting throughout due to shift changes and there was of course no way of knowing who would be on duty when the time came. This worried me, so I began to investigate the alternatives and came across information in a book about the Independent Midwives Association. I followed this up on the internet and began e-mailing some of them and making enquiries. Following this I arranged a meeting with Jo, who was the nearest independant midwife to me. The meeting went really well, and I was convinced straight away that this was what I wanted to do.

My husband, Ian, was a little worried as he had been though a very typical hospital birth with his son from his first marriage. He had found the whole experience stressful and overwhelming and really his impression of labour was quite fearful. Jo was very reassuring and spent a long time answering questions and explaining the various pros and cons of home birth. So, the decision was made and from then on Jo looked after me: no more hospital visits.

I was due to have my baby on 20 November. One week prior to that I was already 4cm dilated and (we thought) ready to go at any time. Jo and I decided we might as well encourage things along so I had been taking homeopathy, using clary sage oil in the bath, going for lots of walks and having sex too – all to try and get things moving.I had also been attending pregnancy yoga classes for eight weeks. And in addition we had three attempts at starting labour with membrane sweeps. Each time I was convinced it was going to start and then nothing happened.

I was beginning to get really fed up and my cervix was dilating more all the time! I had lots of sensations and felt like the baby was going to fall out! I got to seven days overdue and I was panicking that I would soon be forced to go into hospital to be induced and all my plans for an active birth at home, without medical intervention, would be taken out of my hands.

I woke up at eight days overdue at the normal time and when I went to the bathroom had what seemed like a normal period. I hardly dared think that this was it. I had no pains at all so I went back to bed for a bit and kept it to myself. Half an hour later I was sure that this was it and woke Ian. I told him that I thought he should contact Jo and ask her to come (she was an hour's journey away and had said it would progress quickly when it started). I felt so relieved and very excited.

I ran a bath and once in the bath the contractions became intense. I remember trying to find the energy to speak and ask when Jo was arriving; although I still felt very calm it was almost impossible to speak . My dad arrived at this point as we had asked him to be available to organise the pool so that Ian could stay with me. This was a good plan – I needed Ian right by me. After about twenty minutes in the bath I started to feel frightened and like I needed to get out but didn't know how to. I was scared that once out of the water it would be more painful, but I also felt trapped by being in the bath. Ian helped me to get out in between contractions and I lay down on the bathroom floor. I had been there about 5 mins when Jo arrived.

I was very relieved to see Jo and immediately felt calmer as I knew she knew what I wanted and would just take care of things. At this point if I had been in the hands of someone I didn't know it would have been a very different experience.

After a few minutes Jo suggested that we crawl together into the lounge so that I could get into the birth pool. I felt that that was a real challenge but we very slowly crawled together along the hall. It must have looked hilarious from Ian's viewpoint. It seemed to take forever to get there and when I looked at the sides of the pool I felt I'd got to climb Everest to get in. But once in the water it was heaven! It was as though the warm water took all the intensity out of the conractions and made it more managable. I relaxed totally and felt very positive. We had some nice music on and it was snowing outside the window. Being in my own home felt great.

From this point onward things felt quite calm and easy. For the next couple of hours we just kept the water warm and occasionally added some aromatherapy oils. Jo kept checking my blood pressure and the baby's heart rate but did no internal checks as she wanted to just let things go as naturally as possible, and to take our time.

I had been regularly listening to a hypnotherapy CD during pregnancy which was specifically for home birth preparation. I was quite unsure how effective this would be during labour but had enjoyed relaxing to it every evening. When I was actually in labour Jo reminded me that I should maybe listen to it on my headphones and when I did the results were amazing. I went completely into hypnosis and was actually falling asleep in between contractions! Jo told me afterwards that she had never worked with anyone that had used this and that she was astounded at how relaxed and happy I was. I'm really thrilled that I had decided to give this a go and just be open-minded about it.

At about five hours in I was ready to start pushing and was quite shocked by how overwhelming this sensation was. It frightened me, and Jo gave me some Bach flower remedy for fear and anxiety. She also suggested that I change position as up to this point I had been lying on my left side for the whole time in the water and holding Ian's hand. We had planned lots of different positions for labour and practiced them often and yet I had used none of them. So I tried kneeling up leaning on the side of the pool but there was no way that was happening: it was agony! I quickly went back to my left side and decided to stay there. Looking back this was totally not the plan but nothing could have made me change position again!

I found the pushing to be really scary – not agony but just uncomfortable and totally overwhelming. Jo gave me Entonox to use at this point so that I had something to focus my breathing on and this was helpful. The Entonox ran out at one point and I had a little panic but it was soon replaced and I was okay again.

After about an hour of pushing I began to worry that it was never going to happen and I was also worried about whether I would be damaged when the baby did come. I kept saying to Jo, "Will it be all right?" and Ian and Jo were constantly having to reassure me. At this point Ian had been on his knees for six hours or so but every time he tried to go and get a cushion I told him, 'Stay there, don't move!", so he didn't.

Eventually baby Luisa made her appearance still in the water and Ian was really thrilled to see this happen. I think this was great for him and he was really encouraging me all the time saying he could see her and to keep going.

When Jo passed Luisa to me I was so amazed that she was a girl and she looked straight at me and that was an incredible moment. She snuggled up on my chest in the water for ten minutes while we left the cord to stop pulsating. Ian cut the cord and then she sat on his knee wrapped up and she was totally calm and happy. I'm sure that this was another positive part of the home birth expereince as we had lots of time at this point to savour the occassion and look at her and just be together.

I got out of the water and went into the bedroom for the placenta to be delivered as it was slow to happen. Ian sat taking care of Luisa and had a lovely time with her all to himself. I had worried about this stage and heard lots of horrror stories about problems, but it went okay. Then I went and had a lovely shower and got dressed; I even put some mascara on and did my hair! I felt fantastic. Ian and I snuggled up with Luisa and had a lovely time and then my parents came round. Jo stayed with us for a few more hours and then it was just the three of us.

It was wonderful to sleep that night in my own bed with my husband beside me and to have all the comforts of home. I'm sure that it was much nicer for Luisa too. Because I was at home I was much more relaxed. Knowing my midwife really well and building the relationship with her before the birth was really important. The whole experience was totally positive. I feel that I have been very lucky to have exactly the experience of birth that I had hoped for. It was the best experience ever!

Hannah S's story

Fred, 2003

Fred was born the day before our first wedding anniversary and two days before his sister Josie's third birthday. His arrival completed quite a busy hat trick of celebrations!

To understand the reasons behind Fred's home birth option, I feel it is important give a picture of Josie's birth. As soon as Josie decided she was ready to join the world, the contractions began and my body was filled with tension. Although Josie may have been ready, I was not! I kept saying to myself: not just yet, give me a little more time and then I'll be ready.

I curled myself into a foetal position and tried to calm my way out of the pain I was feeling. When I arrived at hospital I was strapped to a device to monitor the baby's heartbeat, which I found very distressing as I waited in anticipation of something being wrong. Hours ticked by and my dilation was very slow. At 2cm dilated, the midwife on call broke my waters, which seemed to increase the ferocity of the contractions. I howled for an epidural and and as soon as this was given I was able to relax and catch up on lost sleep.

As Josie's head was in the wrong position, and the contractions were slow and weak, the doctor overseeing my labour strongly recommended that I have a caesarean, stating that if I was her sister, she'd have me in the operating room straight away. The only reason this did not happen was because of the midwife's steely determination; she quietly stated that although the doctor's opinion was to be respected, she thought I could do it. I have a lot to thank her for, because if she had not been there, it would have been a very different story. Josie was eventually delivered naturally some hours later, and it was amazing to finally hold my little girl in my arms, and breastfeed her for the first time. We had endured a difficult labour, but there was no sense of disappointment. I felt only pride and achievement that despite the high drama, we had come out the other side all safe and healthy.

However, when I began considering Fred's birth plan, I knew I was going to approach it very differently. Leading up to Josie's birth, I had thought as little as I could about the birth itself. I couldn't quite believe that I would be able to push a baby out of my tummy and through the birth canal. When it came to having Fred however, I knew that I could do it and so disbelief at my body's capabilities was not an issue – I had the confidence of experience and was freed to become more attuned to my body's needs.

I wanted the security of a hospital when I gave birth to Josie, and if I had chosen a home birth then, I think I would have found the lack of technology unnerving (although I actually found the hospital technology intimidating and it heightened my sense of fear). Because Josie's labour was long, towards the end, there was an element of clock watching and midwives trying to move the proceedings along. And procedures were perhaps, in retrospect, instigated earlier than need be.

I chose to have a home birth with Fred not because I was against hospital births, but rather because I wanted to deal with the pain and pace of the experience differently. The way I dealt with the labour would obviously impact on this, but I also felt the setting needed to be different and more akin to my pace.

I remember when Fred's labour pains began and the midwife came to visit, she told me how differently midwives view pain as part of childbirth in comparison to the rest of the medical profession. She said that in her experience, doctors generally viewed pain as something to alleviate, because for them, in any other situation, someone in pain would mean that something was wrong. Midwives, however, viewed the pain of contractions as positive: the stronger the contraction pains, the more effective the dilation. I knew that when having Fred, I wanted to try to encompass rather than reject the pain I endured, and to listen to my body's needs and respond appropriately.

My husband, Mark, was very supportive of the decision, although the rest of my family were more concerned than supportive. My parents had both been in the hospital with us when Josie was born, and I think they worried that a second labour would be the same. My mother thought that I had a low pain threshold, but I knew that the many varying factors of Josie's birth must have contributed to the pain I felt.

Fred's labour was very similar to Josie's and the duration was suprisingly long for a second labour: about twenty hours in total. The midwives told me after the event that if it had been an hour longer, I would have ended up in hospital. I would have been fine with this, as I had stated before the birth that my priority was not for Fred to be born at home no matter what, but rather that I was to spend as much time as possible at home, and if that meant Fred was also born at home as well then brilliant!

When Fred's contractions started, my first response was to move about. I had read somewhere that making circular movements in a belly dancer fashion was a useful technique for combating the pain, and I definitely found it helped. I also walked around our neighbourhood – my first walk being at two in the morning.

I had decided that I would pace the coping techniques and interventions used, so that I wasn't rushing through the various pain relief options available and getting to a point where I would then need to opt for a stronger source of pain relief and there-fore have to go to hospital. As soon as the pain reached a certain level and the bellydancing and walking were no longer effective, I attached a TENS machine and continued to walk and belly dance through until about two in the afternoon. I found the TENS machine very effective – I had used a hospital machine when giving birth to Josie, but it was quite old and with a limited choice of levels. I would highly recommend the TENS machine I used for Fred which was hired from a high street chemist.

Mark joined me on my circuits around the local streets, and when the contractions came, I would lean into him until they passed. We must have looked quite a pair, especially when the time lapse between contractions decreased and became more intense. I remember meeting our next-door neighbours in the street and stopping for a chat. When I had a contraction, I'd 'do my thing' while they patiently waited beside me. Once the contraction had gone, we'd carry on chatting!

I also made a point of trying to sleep or at least rest in between my walks. With Josie's birth, I was too tense to relax and almost felt that I couldn't relax too much into sleep as there was "work to be done". This time, I was surprised by the amount of rest I managed in between labour pains.

Another choice I made was to make more noise and groan or howl my way out of the pain. There is a particular noise I still make sometimes to remind Mark of the whole experience. He, however, does not find it that amusing and his normal response is to cover his ears. The neighbourhood did hear much of my groans, but at the time I wasn't bothered by this. It was only afterwards, when I was told that one neighbour nearly called the police as she assumed I was a case of domestic violence, that I was a little embarrassed. But I actually really appreciated the support of the community and was touched by the concern shared and the help we received from neighbours.

As well as my approach being different, the approach the midwives took was also very different: there was no sense of urgency in terms of time. Examinations were kept to a bare minimum and only when necessary. (In hospital with Josie, at one point, internal examinations were every hour.) Monitoring the baby's heartbeat was done with a hand-held monitor every hour or so. The pervading atmosphere was that of calm.

One strong memory I have is of a midwife perched at the end of my bed chatting with me while I sipped on some gas and air. I'd take a gulp and enjoy the intoxicating feeling of floating on the Entonox and when the contraction had stopped we'd continue to chat either about the gossip in my celebrity magazines or about their own birth experiences.

I also had more of a say over whether my waters were broken. They were happy for me to try and deliver Fred complete in the birth sack. However, it got to a point where the contractions were slow and I was getting impatient. At this later point (rather than at 2cm dilated) my waters were broken and I felt a surge of relief. As soon as they were broken, the pushing stage kicked in. They were broken at absolutely the right time, and absolutely at the time I wanted.

The pushing stage involved me on all fours grunting and sipping cups of tea in between pushes. One of the midwives joked that it was one of the most sedate second stages she'd witnessed. Fred was born in the corner of our bedroom. There is still a splatter of blood on the radiator. Mark took Fred into his new bedroom and watched as Fred breathed his first breaths of life and turned from a bluey colour into something more normal, while I was being stitched up. It was all so amazing, yet at the same time felt so normal and calm. At no point was I afraid, and I am sure this was the main factor in my being able to deal with the pain.

When the midwives left, Mark and I got into bed with our new baby snuggled between us. Just the three of us. Such a special and intimate moment, and such a relief that Mark could stay with me rather than leaving me in the birthing suite of a hospital.

Mark felt more involved in Fred's labour than he had with Josie's. He was able to support me through it rather than stand by and watch helplessly. I think this was due partly to him 'knowing the ropes' second time round, but also because he was given the space to be alone with me and become my primary carer.

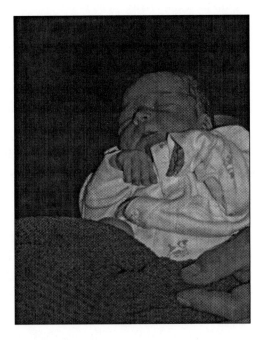

The following day, my parents brought Josie home, and she met Fred in their shared bedroom. She was incredibly matter-of-fact and accepting of her new brother, and I am sure this is in part because her first meeting took place in familiar surroundings. She still remembers the moment vividly. We have a video camera and normally record those special moments, but I'm so glad we didn't record this particular one as it is still very real and clear for Josie. Her memory hasn't morphed into a combination of her real memory and her memory of watching it on video.

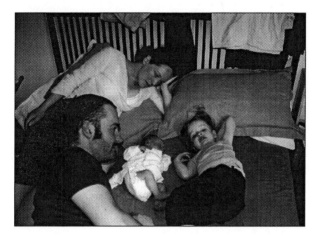

The only regret I have is that we weren't firmer about the amount of visitors later that day and the following day. At least with hospital there were set visiting times, which were short, whereas at home people came and stayed and the house became too chaotic. I should either have stayed in my bed with Fred and left them all to it, or we should have made a point of allowing only a few visitors at a time.

Mark and I built a very strong bond with the midwives and I was very sad when the final visit came and I had to say goodbye. There was a particular midwife who I felt a particularly strong bond for, who on her last visit, brought a present for Josie, which was incredibly touching. The closeness we felt with these midwives was quite amazing: they were involved in such a precious moment of our lives. There is a part of me that wishes I had stayed in touch, but then I also realise the moment was transient and that the connection would never have remained as intense. The experience of the home birth did for a few days make me consider re-training and becoming a midwife, and as I write this, for a flicker of a moment, I am considering it again!

For another perspective on this experience, you can read Mark's story on p.219

Margaret's stories

Caleb, 1972

In 1950 home births were the norm. Nurse Dorrington cycled indefatigably around our area of Cambridge attending mothers at their confinements. I was just one of many children that she helped bring into the world.

When I was pregnant with my first child in 1972 the expectation was that the first child would be born in hospital and any subsequent births might be at home. It was therefore a surprise to my husband and me, and to our family and friends, when our GP made no protest at our request to have a home delivery for our firstborn. Our appointed midwife was delighted, as was her accompanying student who needed to complete her quota of home births before qualifying. They did attend Caleb's birth but it was a close run thing.

The contractions began in the early evening and increased in frequency and intensity quite quickly. We called the duty midwife around midnight. She arrived, accompanied by her student, and began to arrange things to her specification.

We had assembled all the items required in our spare bedroom – rubber sheet, bed pan, nailbrushes, bowls, disinfectant, sheets, towels – but we found that there was something missing. It seemed that we needed eight bricks wrapped in newspaper. Did this mature midwife have a new and different approach to birthing? No, she was not going to risk putting her back out. Our low, single divan needed to be raised to an acceptable height. Dutifully my husband went off into the cold, dark night and found some bricks just down the road where some building work was going on, wrapped them in newspaper as directed and raised the bed. We were young, inexperienced and in the hands of a professional.

As she left the house a couple of hours later she advised us to call our own midwife when she came on duty in the morning. She assured us that nothing would happen before then, gave me something to help me sleep and left. How wrong she was.

When I awoke a few hours later something was definitely happening. By the time I finally roused my husband, who had been sleeping deeply in the next room, it was almost seven o'clock, the time when our own midwife would come on duty. We had no telephone so my husband cycled to the nearest telephone box. If he had gone a hundred yards further he could have knocked on her door, but that didn't seem quite the thing to do at that hour of the morning.

To my relief she and her student arrived promptly and set about delivering my first son who arrived all of a rush just after eight o'clock. As she tidied up and made us comfortable she listened to the tale of our nightime adventures, read the notes and merely commented to her student that her colleague had an old-fashioned way of estimating the progress of labour.

The day passed in a haze of activity centred on our bedroom. The GP arrived to stitch up a small tear and check the baby. The midwives did their job of bathing and weighing the baby, measuring my temperature and tummy and making a late call to check that all was still well. Our mothers lived locally so they were in and out bringing meals, doing washing and admiring their new grandson. When everybody went home I suddenly realised I, who had very little experience of tiny children, was totally responsible for this tiny scrap of humanity. It was quite a shock.

Catriona, 1973

It was a blessing that Caleb was an easy baby and I looked forward to the birth of our next child 18 months later. The same midwife was due to attend accompanied by a different student. Happily she was on duty when we rang for a midwife late one Saturday evening in September.

After such a short first labour she didn't expect to have to wait very long. But as the night drew on the two midwives and my husband sat around my bedside and exhausted every topic of conversation while I laboured on with little sign of progress. Towards dawn my midwife decided something would have to be done. This new baby was facing in the wrong direction. She put on her gloves and set about turning it around. Her intervention did the trick. Labour speeded up and my first daughter was born a little after seven o'clock. My father-in-law used to park his car on our driveway at that time, and as he collected it to go to an early morning church service my husband rushed downstairs to give him the good news.

Later in the day the news was not quite so good. When I was slow to deliver the placenta the student midwife asked if she should give a pull on it. When it came she and the midwife spread it out in our bath. Sadly they concluded that some had been retained and I would need to go to hospital. What I had most feared had happened. I had been trying to avoid hospitalisation and here I was being taken down the road in an ambulance with my newborn baby daughter. It was only a mile but it seemed like the end of the world.

I had the operation that the medical staff assured me was necessary and my daughter spent her first night in the nursery with the other babies. I was told that yes, the baby that I had heard crying during my befuddled sleep was my baby. When the doctor visited later he took pity on me as I could not hold back the tears and agreed that I could be discharged. It was so good to be safely home. Caleb didn't seem to have missed me. He had eyes only for his baby sister whom he had seen so briefly the previous day.

Deborah, 1975

First it had felt a huge responsibility to look after one child; balancing the needs of two small children was an equally big adjustment. When, 15 months later, I was pregnant with my third child I wondered how I should ever manage to look after three children under the age of five. But then something totally unexpected happened. Instead of congratulating me on my good news my mother-in-law told me that the doctors suspected she was pregnant. Within two weeks my children had gained an auntie born prematurely by caesarian section. I carried on, through a trouble-free pregnancy, helping my mother-in law with some of her child care.

Deborah was due to be born at home but as the days overdue added up the doctor began to talk about a hospital delivery.

On a bright September morning I left my two children with their granny in order to attend the busy antenatal clinic. I waited all morning, becoming more and more agitated. It was the last place I wanted to be and I needed to be home with my children. By the time my turn came my blood pressure was understandably high. I could only manage a weak smile when the nurse asked me if I was at all anxious.

After an internal examination the consultant issued his ultimatum of hospitalisation the following day and I stepped out into the hot sun. There was no bus in sight so I set off to walk the mile home, where I found my husband. He had cycled

Margaret's stories

home from work on the other side of town to see how I had
got on.

I had got on better than I thought. I found a show of blood.
My husband stayed at home and it soon became obvious that the
children should go back to their granny's house, ten doors along
the road. We phoned the same midwife from our own house this
time and she soon arrived. By the time my own mother arrived
after tea to hear the news from the hospital (she had no phone)
there were three children, and a new mother peacefully tucked
up in bed. My husband just told her to go upstairs as I was
resting. You can imagine the look of surprise when she found
her new granddaughter by the side of my bed!

Barnabas, 1977

In the summer of 1977 we hoped that our fourth child would
be a Silver Jubillee baby, or at least arrive on his grandfather's
birthday. He was not so obliging. Nor did he arrive at the civilised hour that his next older sister had. We were impressed
by the large, black midwife who came late that June evening
and accurately predicted that he would arrive at two in the
morning.

We were somewhat dumbfounded by the huge amount of
equipment that her student brought in from the car. Our own
midwife normally brought little more than her black bag of
essential equipment. Soon the bedroom was swamped with
packages wrapped in green hospital cloths. Surely the proverbial
kitchen sink must be amongst them!

In spite of all the comings and goings the older children slept
soundly and number four was born weighing in at 9lb 8oz, the
biggest yet. A proper sized baby, commented my mother, who
had produced two similar sized babies.

57

Simeon, 1980

Then the fun began. When I was pregnant with number five, in 1979, my GP decided that he was too out of touch with obstetrics to give medical support. Fewer and fewer mothers were electing to have home births and it had been a long time since he had attended a delivery. He had certainly never been required at one of mine.

Then some astute person noticed that I had had a partially retained placenta after the birth of my second child. This was a very good reason to deliver in hospital. In vain we pointed out that I had delivered two other babies since then without the slightest difficulty. And in vain we tried to convince the medical profession that the partially retained placenta had been caused by an impatient student's intervention.

I was 30 and since I had miscarried the previous year this was my sixth pregnancy. With those factors I was told there might well be complications. I had a different midwife who was practically begging me to give in and go to the maternity hospital. It was, after all, just down the road. All the more reason to start off at home we argued. If anything did go wrong a team could be with us in minutes. But that was selfish, my consultant wrote in a letter to my doctor that was left conveniently unsealed. (This was in the days when patients only got to look at their notes by reading them upside down over the doctor's desk.)

It was then that my new midwife revealed her fear. She had attended a mother with a similar history to mine who had bled to death after the birth. Were we foolish not to heed the medical advice? Were we selfish to insist on an arrangement that helped me to be relaxed? We were not totally irresponsible. We had no intention of insisting on a home delivery at all costs. If complications had arisen during the pregancy I would have gone reluctantly into hospital for mine and the baby's safety.

As the ground floor extension at the back of our house grew steadily that autumn, so did I. I walked the children back and forth to school each day and prepared for Christmas with a new baby. That holiday time was a sort of limbo. Our extension was roofed but awaited the return of the builders to bring it to completion. I awaited the beginning of labour to bring a new member of our family into the world.

In the New Year the builders returned and, to the surprise of the other mothers, I returned, still very pregnant, to the school gate. The medics were not happy. I was healthy but long overdue. We went through the hospital routine once again with the addition of the newly introduced ultrasound scan. For the first time I saw an image of my baby *in utero* on the screen. All looked well. I had a few more days grace.

Deborah remembers going to her granny's and helping her take the chocolate decorations off the Christmas tree the morning that Simeon was born. I remember, on the advice of the midwife who had delivered my last baby, working about the house to keep the contractions going. She and her student sat having a cup of tea with my husband for a while then went off to do a routine post-natal visit. Since she had predicted the timing of the last birth so accurately I had no fear that she would miss the event. Her relaxed attitude and competency born out of long experience gave me confidence. I imagined that the legendary Nurse Dorrington of my childhood would have been like her. Both had seen so many births that nothing would phase them.

When the action moved to our bedroom I was glad that the builders were well out of earshot. Not that the birth was traumatic or noisy. I remember it as being quite civilised in spite of the inherent indignity and messiness of the birthing process.

Feeling a little queasy, I did think that next time I wouldn't eat anything when I was so close to delivery.

Selwyn, 1982

Yes, there was a next time. It was the last and most successful, to my mind. We had had several false alarms with the previous two labours and the same thing seemed to be happening again. So, after lunch on a grey Sunday in March 1982, we wrapped the children up and walked along a footpath through the closest we got to countryside in our locality. The children enjoyed it. We didn't go very far: I didn't want to be too far from the house. After tea I put the children to bed and when they were all safely tucked up at about eight o'clock we called the midwife.

My previous midwife who had been so frightened at the prospect of a sextagravida mother giving birth at home had actually, on her last visit, apologised to me for her negativity. I had only realised how much it had affected me when, on one beautiful sunny day about six months after the birth, I had suddenly realised that I was still alive and had a beautiful healthy baby.

I was not feeling any more than the usual maternal worries about the birth of my last child. When two fully trained midwives arrived that evening I thought it was an indication of the concerns they had about assisting a mother who was pregnant for the seventh time. But we had timed it nicely and within two hours my last and largest baby weighed in at 9lb 12oz. The room was soon tidied up and we were left to get some sleep. When my youngest daughter, aged seven, woke early next morning she was delighted to be called into the bedroom and be the first to see her new baby brother. For older children a home birth seems to be the least disruptive option. Indeed, it is an enriching experience.

Aby's stories

Rosie, 2004

I always knew I would plan to have all my babies at home. In our family (three girls and a boy), we were surrounded by birth from a very early age. Mum was an NCT teacher, so the house was always full of pregnant women and the props associated with teaching natural childbirth – pelvises, dolls, books and diagrams. I was fascinated by every detail. I especially loved the pop-up book where you could gradually open up a woman's body to reveal the foetus curled up and growing inside – magical, mysterious and totally compelling.

When my twin sister and I were four, our brother was born at home, and our Dad recorded the event in a series of photos which are some of the most beautiful pictures I've ever seen. The images have stayed with me through the years and were a huge influence in my decision to train as a midwife. So normal birth was, well, a normal part of everyday life. I'm certain that this awareness of birth as a normal physical process gave me the confidence to believe my body could do it even during the most intense periods of labour.

However, life isn't as simple as all that, and despite planning Rosie's (my first) birth to the last detail, the labour didn't quite follow our nicely laid out plans. My waters broke 48 hours before any contractions started, and while I knew that most women start their labour within 72 hours of their waters breaking, our initial excitement gradually turned to anxiety as the threat of induction in hospital loomed. When contractions did begin it was a relief, and we were really excited to be having our baby at long last.

Twenty-four hours later, however, my cervix still hadn't dilated past 4cm. The contractions were becoming less co-ordinated and were less intense as my body was getting tired. I'd found it hard to eat over the last few hours, and had been upright and swaying what Tom dubbed my 'birth dance' since contractions began, and awake for two days prior to that.

The decision was finally made, with lots of discussion and consideration to our feelings, to transfer into hospital for a bit of help from a hormone drip. My contractions totally stopped as we arrived in hospital – an environment bright and sharp and sterile compared to the cosy, warm, music-filled womb of my living room. Once plugged in and strapped to monitors with wires coming off me like some weird robot, the contractions kicked in again with full force.

I was thankful to have a wonderful midwife who listened to my wishes to achieve an active labour despite the drip, baby monitor and IV antibiotics. I can still picture the look on the junior doctor's face as she said, "I'm told you don't want an epidural… How will you cope with the pain?!" But I knew I wanted my body in full working order. Nobody was going to take this experience away from me: I'd been looking forward to it for years.

I remained upright throughout, hanging off Tom for dear life, and after squatting for 45 minutes of pushing Rosie was finally born. We were totally exhausted, but utterly elated to meet our baby daughter, all pink and amazing. I felt about ten feet tall having given birth actively despite all the interventions. I'm certain that having planned a home birth and focused on normal labour for so long I felt more able to assert my wishes once I'd moved into the hospital environment.

I daydreamed about every detail of her birth for weeks and months afterwards, remembering it all with such a warm glow and sense of amazement at what I'd done. Such beautiful memories.

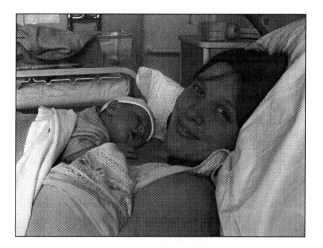

It was such a satisfying experience, particularly afterwards when, to my total surprise, I had my sex drive back almost immediately. And when we did make love again it was as though my whole body worked better. No one tells you that sex can get better after having a baby – what a revelation!

Bede, 2005

I fell pregnant again, to our delight, when Rosie was six months old. And once again I planned a home birth. Inevitably we looked forward to Bede's birth with slightly less certainty that all would go to plan. This was borne out when, on a routine antenatal visit on my due date, the doctor suspected he might be breech and we were sent off to hospital for a scan. Sure enough he was happily sitting with his feet in my pelvis, and we were offered an ECV (external cephalic version), where they manually turn the baby. Suddenly our approaching birth wasn't quite so simple, and I saw my vision of a water birth at home drifting out of reach.

We had to consider the fact that he might remain breech, in which case we were facing either a vaginal breech delivery (my first choice) or, if it came to it, an emergency C-section. They mentioned an elective C-section, but there seemed so many other avenues to try first that I didn't really consider it. Our biggest hope lay in the baby turning and staying turned.

A senior midwife performed the procedure, which felt like an incredibly strong tummy massage. She found the baby's head and bum, grabbed hold and pulled and pushed as hard as she could. It was uncomfortable but not painful and I was desperate to try anything that might win me back my coveted home birth.

It is the most incredible sensation, having a baby turned a full circle inside you. Three times she tried, three times his head swung straight back round to the top of my tummy. Until finally she laid her hands over mine and we both bore down together as hard as we possibly could and he blessedly stayed. What an achievement! My planned birth swung back into view again.

I was sent home with an appointment to return for a further scan the next day to check he'd stayed. Then I spent an anxious 24 hours convinced he'd turned again – I hardly dared to lie down in case he did. But on scan we immediately saw his head nestled happily in my pelvis and I literally danced all the way back to the car with happiness, a ridiculous grin on my face. Such a minor intervention to avoid such a major one – I'd recommend the procedure to anyone.

I had a show three days later, on a Saturday morning in mid-September. I began to have mild contractions that evening, and called Mum over to stay in case she was needed to look after Rosie that night, and we set the pool up so we were all ready. It was a long slow night after that, with not very much happening, and after a 3am trek round the neighbourhood to see if we could get things going, we finally decided to try and salvage what was left of the night and get some rest.

We took Rosie out for a long walk in the park the next day and I had occasional twinges every hour or so, but began to feel a bit silly for having got all excited and put the pool up already. It filled the kitchen, and since it could be some days before anything happened again I realised it could seriously start to get in the way!

That evening after Rosie had gone to bed Tom and I had sex, partly as we knew it might not happen again for a while if the baby was coming, and partly because we knew it might actually help the baby to arive. Rosie had been ten days overdue, so I expected a bit of a wait this time too.

Lo and behold, my waters broke not long afterwards. I had actually just answered the phone to a friend when I felt a strong twangy pop and gave a little yelp as I realised my waters had gone. I got off the phone fairly quickly and called my sister to let her know, and started to get excited with Tom. We were fairly cautious this time knowing it had taken two days for anything to happen with Rosie, so I was really pleased to feel the first contractions start shortly after.

From then on we spent a frustrating night, with contractions coming and going at some cosmic whim. It's hard to be totally rational about a slow start to labour even though you know all is well. And I admit that by Monday morning I was feeling pretty demoralised. I was disappointed to feel so negative about being in labour, but I knew it was because it reminded me of the hours of slow progress with Rosie before I needed to move to hospital.

However, I had to remind myself I wasn't even in established labour yet (the midwife had checked me after my waters went: 2cm dilated and contracting roughly every ten minutes does not constitute 'real' labour, but it blooming well feels like it!). No ticking clock to check me against yet, which was good, although we had spent two nights up and about so were pretty tired which wasn't so good.

Rosie had woken on Monday morning, had her morning milk with us as usual and then been collected by grandma who was looking after her for the day so that we could either have this baby or get some much needed rest. I didn't have any objections to Rosie seeing me give birth, but I did think it might be a bit distracting for me, having to focus on her needs too.

By 10am, after a bit of a doze, the contractions started to come regularly again every ten minutes, and they felt like they meant business this time. We phoned the on-call midwife who turned out to be Sue, someone I'd worked with during my training, so we already had an easy relationship with each other. I was so pleased to have someone I knew with me. We established that I was 3cm dilated at this point and the baby's head was still quite high, which may have explained the slowish progress, but all the signs were good. She left me in a confident mood, reminding me that she had a clinic until 4pm, but to call someone earlier if I needed them.

Time went on. Tom and I played Trivial Pursuit while I tried to handle contractions the way I had last time – upright and swaying. It wasn't working as well as it had with Rosie; it just didn't feel as right somehow. Then out of sheer tiredness more than anything I moved onto the floor, kneeling on a cot mattress and resting my body, arms and head on the birth ball. Finally I seemed to have found the right position.

With the rolling of the ball my body moved in all the ways it needed to during the contractions that suddenly started coming every five minutes. No gradual change, just bang into full-on labour! Even my noises changed and I started lowing like a cow – lower and longer with each tightening. It was around 4pm now and I remember noticing the neighbour's kids coming home from school and wondering what they'd make of the noises (incredibly they tell me they didn't hear a thing!).

Every detail of this labour is so vivid: as I was using only the TENS machine and Tom's massage to help me I wasn't at all spaced out during contractions. And Tom and I definitely felt like we'd got into the groove together, especially now that he could actively help me by pressing on my lower back. We became a real team.

As I really wanted it to be Sue who was with me during the birth and she'd said she was busy until 4pm I didn't call until then, by which point I really *did* want her to be there with me. Luckily, I had had a sudden, random urge for orange ice-lollies eartlier and had sent Verity out on a mission to get me some, (a definite advantage of home birth!), so she arrived just around this time and was a really reassuring presence.

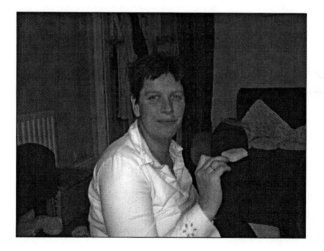

I realised how important it was for me to have another woman around. My mum had been there at Rosie's birth and when Verity arrived I realised what had been missing from the equation. Tom was wonderful, but we were such a team by this point that I needed someone slightly more removed from the event to be of more practical help and support. The pool needed topping up with hot water and I wasn't letting Tom out of my sight!

Just as Verity turned up I had three socking great contractions really close together and asked Tom to call Sue again and let her know I'd really appreciate her being there *now*. Internally I actually thought I was getting close to pushing with those last few contractions and didn't want to be alone any longer.

In retrospect I realise I should have called someone out earlier because I did feel very vulnerable being in quite strong labour with no midwife around. But then, I hadn't expected things to move on quite so quickly once the contractions actually got going. What a change from last time.

When Sue arrived around 5pm, she seemed to spend an eternity unloading all her stuff, phoning her kids to let them know she'd be home late, calling the second midwife… while I was gagging either for some gas and air or for her to get on and do an internal so I could use the pool.

I was so hopeful I'd actually get to use the water this time around, and thought I must be several centimetres dilated by this point – going by the 'pushy' feelings I was getting, I thought at least seven or eight. She finally examined me at about quarter past five, on the living room floor, and said I was 5cm but very stretchy. I didn't actually believe her but 5cm was enough to get me in the pool, so I was fine with that.

I asked again for some gas and air, but Sue suggested I try the water on its own first to see how I got on, so I took the TENS machine off and handed it to Tom. In my haste to climb into the pool before another contraction hit I forgot to turn it off: the sticky pads stuck to his hand and he got the shock of his life! Still giggling, I made it into the water, and into absolute heaven.

I never would have believed warm water could feel so amazingly good. I got on my hands and knees as before then just stretched my legs right out behind me and floated. It was utterly wonderful to have the buoyancy and freedom of space and movement, and I instantly relaxed. Tom tried once to press my lower back like before but I didn't need him to anymore. All of the pressure had eased with the warmth of the water. It was total bliss.

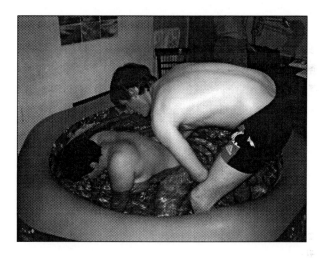

After only a couple more contractions I knew things were really happening fast, so I felt inside and there was the head, just sitting in the birth canal. Looking back I think the rocking motion of my hips as I climbed into the pool must have just slotted his head right down into my pelvis and onto the cervix, and that combined with the total relaxation of getting into the water must have dilated me virtually immediately the rest of the way to 10cm. It happened in the space of about ten minutes.

I said I could feel the head, but nobody seemed too alarmed: Sue carried on getting her gear ready somewhere off to the side of the pool out of sight. So I just got on with it. I knew he was coming really fast now, and said so. I distinctly remember thinking I should let everyone know what was happening in case they didn't realise!

I was trying really hard not to bear down, which is so instinctive on hands and knees. I wanted to birth this baby nice and gently. Tom suggested I turned onto my back to slow the pushing reflex down which was a great idea. He sat behind me and supported me as I tried to concentrate on not actively pushing. I tried to keep my mouth open and relaxed and could feel the head moving all the way down as he was squeezed out of his own accord. I put my hand down and guided him out as the head crowned, and felt amazed that I was doing it all on my own. No midwife's hands, just mine touching my baby's head for the first time.

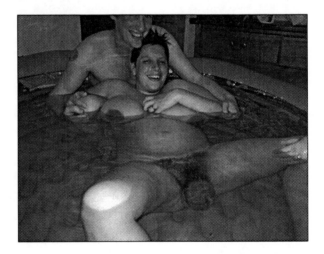

We had a few minutes rest then, Tom and I looking and wondering at this baby's head just sitting there between my legs under water: what an incredible sight! Then at 5:45pm, just thirty minutes after climbing into the pool, Tom reached down and pulled him out and onto me and we discovered we had a beautiful boy. What a lovely surprise.

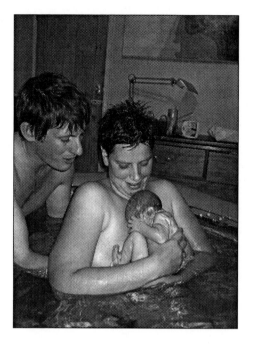

Verity, who had firmly placed herself at the business end of things so as not to miss out on a moment of the action, rushed off to fetch Rosie to meet her little brother and five minutes later my daughter, Mum, brother and nephew all crowded around the pool to welcome Bede. It was such a fantastic family occasion – Mum burst into tears as soon as she walked into the room and when I asked her why she replied it was because we just looked so peaceful, which I thought was a perfect description of how we felt, sitting there in our little pool of calm.

After putting Bede to the breast to help the placenta come I climbed out of the pool, squatted for another small push and the birth was over. Sue gave me a quick check to see if I'd torn; I'd felt already and knew I was fine – in fact I virtually didn't feel anything, no soreness, nothing. I felt, incredibly, as though I'd just had sex rather than a baby. What a revelation: my God, our bodies really are made to do this!

Bede was very conveniently born just before Rosie's bedtime, so Mum took her upstairs and gave her the normal bath time, then Tom gave her a story and milk before rejoining us as we started the celebrations.

We moved to the living room, Bede nestled against my skin, and sat sipping champagne and quietly digesting the fact of a new life. Verity popped home and reappeared a while later with food. I realised I was ravenous and ate two whole plates of shepherds pie, the tastiest pie I've ever eaten! And once the midwives had done their final checks, collected their gear and said goodbye, we said goodnight to the family and headed upstairs to bed.

For another perspective on this experience, you can read Tom's story on p.237

Patricia's story

George, 2003

When I became pregnant with my first child there was never any question in my mind that I wanted a home birth. My experiences of the medical profession through the years were, on the whole, negative ones. I felt that I had been judged, treated with insensitivity, given inappropriate health care and rarely respected for having knowledge about my own health. I also mistrusted the techniques and approaches of the mainstream medical profession towards childbirth. I believe that common practices in this field are flawed, and take control of the birth away from the mother.

One way in which I believe this form of control manifestes itself is in the use of drugs during birth. I find it hypocritical that, for example, strong opiate-based substances can be given to a women during one of the most dangerous times of her life, a time when she needs all her faculties intact. How can a woman say what she wants if she is zoned out on some heroin-like substance? She can't. I also suspected that drugs used during birth stay in the system and affect the child afterwards.

My basic knowledge of yoga made me realise that some of the conventional positions in which to give birth are silly and defy gravity. At the same time I believe that nature knows how to create babies without loads of medical intervention: a hospital birth did not match up with this belief. I was far more scared of going to hospital than of having a baby at home. I wanted to retain as much control over the birth as possible; being in my own space was essential to that.

Thinking back, my midwives were very supportive of my desire for a home birth. They seemed excited about the prospect of delivering a child this way. I can't remember what my dad thought about my decision but my mum described me as 'mad' for wanting to do things this way. Obviously this didn't make my pregnancy any easier, but I was expecting this reaction from people.

I think my partner, Bill, understood my reasons for wanting a home birth and he completely supported my decision. What he didn't do was become actively involved in the preparations. I was disappointed that he didn't share this with me, particularly considering he was to be my birth partner, but his mind was on other things. We were travelling (technically homeless) when I conceived, with little money. The pregnancy was spent finding a house, decorating it, getting to know the area and earning money.

I was nearly two weeks overdue, and booked into the hospital to be persuaded into an induction when my labour started. With hindsight I realise the labour actually built up slowly over a number of days, with a gradual build up of pain around my pelvic region. There were occasional sharper, more localised pains, too, but one morning I woke up and the pains were noticeably stronger.

The labour seemed to be building through the morning: a friend came over for tea and I remember telling her that I thought I'd be having the baby that day. I think she thought I was joking. At about 11:00am Bill's friend came round to visit, and we all agreed to take the dog for a walk. I was determined to keep upright and moving for as long as possible. I went upstairs and then some pain really hit me. I shouted to Bill and told him I didn't think I would be going out for a walk. We decided to telephone the on-call midwife.

Because of the support I had had from my midwives I was not prepared for the reaction on the other end of the phone. I explained that my contractions had started and gave my name. The woman at the other end of the phone told me to go to the hospital. I explained that I was going to have a home birth, and she replied something along the lines of "Oh dear".

Despite my normal midwife being well aware of the fact that I was due for one, this lady did not know that a home birth was imminent. This was not exactly reassuring. Anyway, she told me that she was too busy to come over immediately but would be over in a few hours. At this stage I contacted a woman I had been introduced to, who was also a midwife, to let her know what was going on. I called her with no expectations: she said she would come over to see me.

By this stage my contractions had become very painful, although not that frequent. They were scaring me. I was shocked by their intensity and remember saying to Bill, "They shouldn't be like this."

After an hour or so of the occasional very distressing and painful contraction my midwife friend, Charlotte, appeared. I had now retreated to my bedroom where I intended to have my baby. I can't remember what I was doing at this point, but she talked me through the contractions I was experiencing. She was extremely encouraging and told me I was doing well. This had the effect of making me feel more relaxed about what was happening.

I'm not sure exactly when the official midwife came around, sometime around three o'clock. As soon as I saw her, I knew who she was by the way she was dressed. My friend had had a difficult home birth with this particular midwife (they had clashed towards the end of the birth) and had described her to me.

She looked at my notes, felt my tummy and did an internal. She then told me a number of things. Firstly she told me that my iron levels were too low for a home birth, although I was not anaemic. She told me that she thought I was not coping with the labour pains very well. My baby was lying back to back, not the best position to give birth. She said I would have a long and painful labour and that I would lose a lot of blood. She said she wanted me to go to the hospital for the birth.

Charlotte was downstairs as she was not present on a professional basis. I didn't agree with the midwife, particularly over the iron issue because this would have been mentioned to me before if it had been a problem. She called Charlotte up so that we could discuss the issues. Charlotte stated that these were no reasons to send me to hospital, so I decided to stay at home. The official midwife left, saying that she would be back in a few hours and the decision as to whether I would birth at home would be taken then.

As soon as she left, Charlotte appeared to have a new sense of urgency about her. She asked Bill to bring a chair from downstairs and got me to sit on it, facing the back of the seat. For a large part of the next few hours I sat on this chair. Occasionally I would get down, and instinctively went into different positions to deal with the pain. For example going on all fours with my head down and bum in the air. I realise now that sometimes I was attempting to reduce the pain. Charlotte wouldn't let me do this for long though, and would have me back on the chair, ensuring that I was bringing on the labour by allowing the babies head to put pressure onto my cervix.

The pains were building in intensity, both Charlotte and Bill were supporting me with encouraging words and reminding me to use my breath to deal with the pain of labour. Charlotte massaged my back with a combination of essential oils, which included jasmine and clary sage. These helped to relax me but also encouraged the contractions.

By now I had lost all concept of time. What I concentrated on was dealing with the contractions and resting in between. I took some fluids and ate a little yoghurt and honey between contractions. Honey is an excellent source of sugars, of a type which can be absorbed easily by the body. I felt immediate benefit from eating: it gave me more energy to deal with the labour.

The combination of pain and chemicals being released in my body was definitely taking me to another state. The contractions just gradually increased in their intensity, slowly building up my tolerance to prepare me for the birth. As I had asked him to, Bill reminded me during the more painful moments that the pain would not last forever, and this really helped.

Meditation, which I learnt when I was younger, had taught me to observe the pain, not to fight it, and this helped me to relax into the contractions. Focused breathing was essential and my practice of yoga meant that this came to me instinctively. All the time though, in the back of my mind, was the question of whether I would have my child at home.

I think around seven o'clock the midwife returned. She checked me internally and immediately her demeanour changed: my cervix had opened a lot. We were going ahead with the home birth. Charlotte left at this stage, and I remember her saying it was to let me have my own time, or something like that.

Bill looked tired and stressed out. He had been a general skivvy, making cups of tea, and bringing equipment up from the midwife's car. With Charlotte out of the way he really began to take on the role of birth partner. He must have been learning from Charlotte and without her presence was able to get more involved. He massaged my back, held me and said the right things to encourage me through the contractions. The midwife had very quickly called for back up, so we waited for number two midwife to assist in the final stages.

I think by this stage I was completely naked apart from a knee-high pair of stripy socks, which I insisted on wearing.

Somehow I gained some amusement from this. My waters had not broken, and the midwife wanted to break them. I refused, as I still wanted as few interventions as possible. Instead, she told me to go to the toilet. I remember hanging from our toilet door shouting for Bill because I was experiencing the most intense contraction. My waters had broken, but not completely. A bag of fluid, like a condom full of water, was swinging from between my legs. The midwife burst it – another comedy moment.

Around this time the second midwife arrived and it was time to give birth! I wanted to do this squatting, but needed a hard surface to squat on, the floor. The midwife would not allow this. She said the baby might hit the floor when I gave birth. I was too weak and overcome by contractions to argue, but was not happy about this. We ended up in a position with Bill supporting me from behind, with my bum resting on the edge of our futon. This allowed the midwife to see what was going on, and at least I wasn't lying down.

The birth itself was, of course, even more painful. My baby was turning into the correct position as it moved down and out. Bill said that I went very pale. I don't really remember that much about it. Just that I relied completely on what my midwife told me to do, and, despite all the other issues I had had with her, she did a brilliant job.

Just when I felt I had no strength left to push, out popped a little boy. Quickly he was placed on my chest and, as I had requested, the cord was not immediately cut. When it was finally cut the other midwife took my baby and put some clothes on him with Bill's help.

I still had to birth the placenta, which was also done naturally. I remember such an intense desire to take my son back into my arms at this at this stage, and couldn't wait to have him back. He did not breastfeed immediately, but the midwives said not to worry about that. They encouraged me to keep him in bed with me that night, and left saying what a wonderful birth it had been.

It was definitely the most amazing experience I had ever had and I was high from that for a while after the birth. I also felt stronger and more capable, because I had managed to cope without using any drugs. This experience had reinforced my belief in women's instinctive ability to give birth: it is a natural thing to do.

We were left alone with our baby. I now was in my own space where I had the freedom to learn to look after my child without other people interfering. The midwives had told me that I was one of the most polite women they had ever helped to give birth. I think this was because I was at home where I felt comfortable and could fully concentrate on my labour. My body had released some very helpful chemicals too, and these hadn't been masked by the use of pharmaceutical drugs.

I did eventually complain about some aspects of the care I received during my labour. These were dealt with, but it left me with very mixed feelings. My decision to complain had repercussions for me during my next pregnancy and birth experience, but that is another story.

Sarah S's stories

Max, 1995

I don't remember consciously deciding to have a home birth; I think I just assumed that I would. My sister had had two lovely home births and a friend (although far away in Bath) had just had a lovely one too. When I was newly pregnant she sent me a book she had used called *Active Birth*, by Janet Balaskas, which was brilliant. It was the first, and only, 'birth' book that I read and it just made sense.

As long as everything was okay (and I would have gone into hospital had I really felt the baby was at risk) home was the best place for me, the baby and my husband. I have a fear of hospitals and I really felt that if I did go into hospital I would be so tense that nothing would come out!

I felt very strongly that I wanted my partner to be involved during the birth and especially afterwards, that he and we needed time to bond together. I had heard stories of fathers being sent home after the birth of their children because it hadn't been during visiting hours which still appals me: it is such a special time for all the family.

I also assumed that it would be fairly easy to have a home birth, even with a first child, and in some senses it was. My midwife was fantastic (and I think quite excited by it too) and a strong believer in home births, although I had been ready to change midwives if she didn't support me. My friend had given me the number of the 'radical midwives' who could put me in touch with a midwife who could help. With such an excellent name, I was a bit disappointed not to meet any!

Sarah S's stories

My husband was very supportive too and I don't know whether I would have had a home birth without this. Although I felt like a home birth was the most natural and obvious choice, I also think it's important that both parents are involved and happy with the birth choice.

My doctor, however, was very nervous about it all and tried many times (both openly and covertly) to dissuade me. These attempts largely went over my head, since the midwife used to read out the concerns that he had written on my notes and laugh about them with me.

A few weeks before I was due my doctor sent me for a scan as he was 'concerned' about the size of the baby. For this first scan the doctor had written a note to the consultant asking him to 'dissuade this young lady from having a home birth'. He didn't, despite his best attempts, and the scan was fine.

A week before I gave birth the doctor told me during a routine check that he thought I might be having twins! He also gave me the 'a handicapped baby is for life' talk, which I must admit was the first time I felt anxious about our decision. My husband and I had already talked about the real, though small, possibility that if the baby needed significant medical attention it wouldn't get it immediately (we were ten minutes away from the hospital) but that, sad though it is, it might be better to let nature take its course. We accepted that 'natural' can also mean the side of nature it would be nice to forget, that of death rather than 'life at all cost'.

Having been unswayed by any of the doctor's obstructions, he did on my last visit seem to accept my decision and actually spent a long time with me talking about breathing and relaxation during birth. The advice really helped and I was touched that in the end he was supportive.

There was a mixed reaction from family and friends, but again their concerns largely washed over me, especially those of

81

pregnant friends. I was equally concerned about them being in the hands of hospital staff, which to me was much more frightening. I was nervous about the birth but not really my choice for a home birth which I always felt was the right choice for me. If I felt people were going to be negative about my choice, often I kept quiet rather than have to explain myself. I tended to talk only in depth about my concerns about birth to those who I knew would be supportive and talk positively about giving birth.

The antenatal classes were something else, though, and I still feel passionately angry about them today, ten years later. The midwife leading the classes introduced birth as, "the most painful thing you can imagine times one thousand," and declared that all women should have an epidural. There was no talk of active birth, or of any birth positions other than that of lying down, which seemed archaic to me after reading Balaskas and having some understanding of the physiology of birth.

In the 'circle discussion time', when I said I hoped for a home birth the midwife moved swiftly on to the next person! At our reunion, while sharing our birth stories, I quietly said that I had had a lovely home birth and that everything was fine. Again, she moved swiftly onto the next person, lingering on all the worst and most painful experiences. It seems sad that there is such a negative attitude to birth right from the beginning, especially with new and already anxious mothers.

Max came two weeks early so I didn't have time to dwell on it too much and was only just in the time limit allowed for a home birth (phew!). I was in labour for a few days I think, having contractions on and off. I sort of ignored it, not admitting it to myself and not really knowing for sure as he was my first and there was nothing to measure it against. I thought that if people started fussing I wouldn't be able to handle it. I even skipped the antenatal class on the Friday, as I was scared that someone might notice and they would make me have the baby there at the hospital!

On the Saturday night we stayed up late – playing golf in a neighbour's flat of all things. When we got home at about eleven o'clock (the latest I had stayed up in months) I waited until Lorenzo, my husband, had gone to bed then put a film on, and by this time couldn't sit down with the pain. I had been told in the antenatal class to be prepared for a long labour and to snack in early labour, so I ate hot cross buns standing up.

The contractions were about a minute apart and I really don't know why I kept it secret for so long. Even when I phoned the midwife I said the contractions were about ten minutes apart. I thought she just wouldn't believe me and I still wasn't really sure if this was labour. I also really didn't want anyone near me fussing or panicking. I read afterwards that often cows find a quiet corner of a barn to give birth in on their own and this was really how it felt.

I woke Lorenzo up as the pain was getting too much. By the time the midwife came I was taking what I now know is my most comfortable birth position – on the toilet. I had diarrhoea and sickness together for what seemed like ages. I regretted those hot cross buns, but I was so glad I wasn't in a hospital. Being on my own in the loo with a sick bowl, with the midwife and Lorenzo in the other room was just fine.

After a while (once emptied) I went into the lounge with gas and air and towards six o clock the pain became too much. I asked for pethidine, which I was given. I hadn't had an internal exam to see how far dilated I was (and never did have in my two subsequent labours) and I think it was assumed that I still had a long labour to go. I gave birth an hour later which meant that my lovely son, Max, was very sleepy and didn't feed properly.

I had tremendous trouble feeding him and I always wondered whether, if I had known how far gone I was, I would have been able to carry on without pethindine. I was also unaware of the effect it has on the baby, if given so close to birth.

The actual birth is a bit blurry as a result of the pethidine; he was very quick down the birth canal and I gave birth in the supported squatting position, holding Lorenzo. It came as a surprise to the midwife and Lorenzo, who were busy chatting, so there was only one midwife present at the birth. The other arrived in time for me to give birth to the placenta which I had wanted to do naturally. I remember being fascinated by how big and amazing it was.

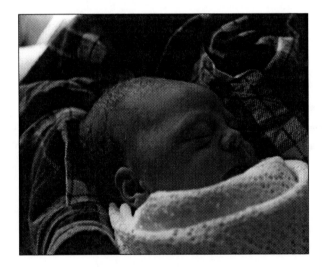

Max was just gorgeous; I really couldn't sleep for days afterwards, I felt so overwhelmed with protectiveness. I had given birth at around 7.00am, so the full-on labour had only been about eight hours. Lorenzo went over to our friend's flat across the corridor where we had been playing golf the night before (she was also pregnant and thought the idea of home birth was just too much) saying, "We've got something to show you." I will never forget her face as she walked in to find me on a plastic sheet on the floor with a baby and probably lots of other messy stuff we were just too elated to notice.

After the birth, I don't feel I always got the rest I needed: being at home, I wanted to carry on as normal and it was more difficult to manage visits. I found feeding so difficult. I had a very sleepy baby and was so engorged. I am not sure whether being in a hospital would have solved these things but it did mean I had to be proactive in finding help. After a midwife told me I would never be able to breastfeed, I found a wonderful breast-feeding counsellor who taught me, after a few tearful visits to her house, how to feed properly, something I am so thankful for.

Nathaniel, 1998

When I was pregnant again, I didn't even think about having a hospital birth. At the time I was so busy and tired from looking after my three year old and doing a job I hated. I remember waking up on the morning he was born thinking 'I hope I don't give birth today' as I really didn't feel I had the mental energy.

As I got up, I found that I had had a show but again did my best to ignore labour. My husband went to work; I took my son to toddler group. I told my close friend, Carol, who was lined up to look after Max, and she came back for a cup of tea while I carried on pretending I was fine. At about 10:30 though, I had to tell Carol to call the midwife and get Lorenzo back from work.

Although it was mentioned on the birth plan that I had had a quick labour previously, the midwife came and went, saying she would be back later. Things went so quickly from then on. My husband was wonderful. I was on the toilet again for the whole time with sickness and diarrhoea and when I started shouting a sort of guttural, pushing shout, Lorenzo (thank God) went and phoned the midwife who was sitting down the road in her car.

She came in and was trying to set up the gas and air before she came upstairs. The baby was coming down the birth canal and I was pushing and shouting, unaware of anyone or anything else, completely overtaken by the pain and the instinct to push. Lorenzo must have been able to tell – he called the midwife to "Get up here!" just as Nathaniel's head was crowning.

The cord was around his neck and it still gets me inside thinking about what might have happened if it had just been me and Lorenzo as I really was oblivious to anything other than what my body was telling me to do, which was to push.

My gorgeous son was born with a very messy splash on the bathroom floor! After the birth it took me a long time to recover. It was so quick and I was so concerned about Max, that he would be okay. I also wasn't very good at asking for help. My husband went to work two days later and I struggled to look after the two children.

I was still in shock and physically worn out. My health visitor was useless, handing me a leaflet on post-natal depression rather than talking practically about help. I think the shock of a quick labour – waking up pregnant then having a baby in my arms by lunchtime – together with very little help and rest in the months after birth, meant that it took me a long time to recover mentally and physically. I still find it upsetting to think about this second birth. I had friends who had gone into the local hospital's 'hotel' after their hospital births and wished that I felt able to have a baby in hospital so that I could have had a proper rest afterwards.

Isaac, 2002

When I was pregnant for a third time I planned much more carefully for the time after the birth. I worked many extra hours so that we could afford for Lorenzo to have a month off work. I saw a homeopath early on in pregnancy which helped with the morning sickness that I had had in the previous pregnancies. Working this time in a job I enjoyed in many ways gave me the 'rest' I needed. So all these together meant that I felt generally less tired when it came to the birth.

I couldn't have asked for a more wonderful midwife for the birth. She was Jamaican and this was her last birth before she retired. Her main role was looking after pregnant teenage girls so she was very caring and nurturing towards me. I remember sitting on the toilet seat afterwards, wrapped in towels, while she dried in-between my toes. When I told her how lovely it was she said it was probably the last time I was going to be looked after for a while and that she did if for all her 'girls'. Just wonderful.

She wasn't impressed, though, with the thought of me having a baby in the bathroom (it was only a little room). Lorenzo, on her arrival, had taken her into the lounge and told her she wasn't allowed to leave and to listen to him before she was allowed upstairs! I was, of course, already on the toilet by this time. She did try to give me an internal and to guide me to the bedroom but I just couldn't.

The labour was so intense and I knew how the pattern of labour was going to be. I did manage to have some gas and air this time which was wonderful; Lorenzo even had some. After one and a half hours labour, all on the toilet, Isaac was born on the bathroom floor. I can still hear the midwife saying resign-edly, "Okay, have it in the bathroom then."

Afterwards, she washed me and tucked me, Lorenzo and my lovely son Isaac into bed before going down to write her notes. The second midwife came an hour or so later, and as she walked in our bedroom said, "Oh wow, my nephew was born in this room, this is such a happy house!" which was just lovely. It did feel so special to have the children actually born in our house.

I didn't come downstairs for about a week – I had learnt from the last time! My new health visitor was wonderful and encouraged me to take all the help that I could, something I hadn't felt able to do last time. She would come round and make me a cup of tea and play with Nathaniel, which was just the best help ever. I had days of exhaustion but nothing like before.

Looking back, I feel like my experience of home birth has been very mixed. The overriding thing for me is that through all three of them it was very much myself and my husband having the baby. We did it together with the help of a midwife and I couldn't imagine anything different. I wouldn't want it to be any other way. All three births were special experiences I shall treasure forever.

Sarah W's story

Abigail, 2005

My name is Sarah. I am 31 years old and I live in Bingham with my husband, Ted, and our two daughters, Emily and Abigail. This is our story of bringing Abigail into the world at home and what an incredible experience it was.

We moved to Bingham in 2004 and I found out that I was pregnant two weeks after moving house. We were over the moon but I was apprehensive, as I didn't know the local health centre and team of midwives. Having had a normal, nine-hour delivery with Emily, I knew that I wanted to try and have my second baby at home.

I didn't know how my husband, family, friends or the community midwives would react. When I spoke to my husband about it, he said "Okay," but wanted to know the facts and find out as much information as possible. He was not especially keen due to the distance we lived from the hospital (about 45 minutes) and the risks associated with childbirth. I decided to wait until my ten-week appointment with the midwife and ask her what she thought.

At the appointment my midwife, Jackie, told me that I was a perfect candidate for a home birth as my labour with Emily had been so straightforward. She did say that she would prefer me to have my baby in hospital but also that she would support me if I wanted to do it at home. I was quite surprised at her attitude; I had thought I was going to have to put up a fight to get what I wanted.

Jackie would come to my home and speak to Ted and me and I didn't have to make a decision until I was 32 weeks pregnant.

This gave me time to do some research and make my choice. I also felt that it wasn't just my decision to make. I had to take into account my husband's views and what would be best for Emily.

As I went through my pregnancy I spoke to my friends and family about what they thought of me having a home birth. My best friend told me that she thought it was up to me and if I wanted to do it that I should go for it. She said, "If there is anyone strong enough to cope with birth at home, it is you Sarah." She was really positive and supportive.

Some were concerned. They thought I was crazy for even thinking of doing it at home. However, other friends and family who know me very well offered words of support. Everyone just wanted the baby and me to be as safe as possible. The one thing I couldn't explain to them was the feeling inside me that it felt so right. I just wanted to have my baby at home and I felt I was confident enough to do it.

When Jackie came to see Ted and me at home, I had a list of questions to ask. Who would be there during labour and for how long? What preparation was required in terms of where to have the baby? What medical equipment would be needed for pain relief, monitoring the baby's heart rate, Apgar tests, stitches and so on? How much mess would be involved? Was I likely to have a similar labour to my previous one? And was I likely to have my baby early as with Emily?

I also wanted to know about the risks to me and my baby. What happens if something goes wrong? How long will the midwives stay afterwards? When will the doctor come? What happens about the hearing tests and paediatric tests they do in hospital?

Jackie was really thorough and made me feel very comfortable about having my baby at home. I was keen for her to deliver, as I felt confident with her. I liked her approach: strong, direct and very capable. I needed someone who could handle the pressure!

Ted felt more positive about the idea but he still wanted me to go to hospital due to the risks. We discussed it at length and had some time to think about it before making our final decision. Ted told me that if I wanted to have our baby at home he would support me 100%, but that his personal preference would be for the hospital.

I knew that I wanted to give it a go, and when I told Jackie she reminded me that I could always change my mind and go into hospital at any point. I felt really happy with this situation, as I didn't know how I was going to feel once I was in labour. I have always felt that labour should be viewed in an ever-changing way. You need to go with the flow, as you just don't know how your body or the baby is going to react. You should therefore have a positive and open approach to the 'job in hand'.

Jackie told me that she would put the relevant paperwork in place, gave me a list of things that I needed for labour at home and told me she would visit to see what I had collected and which room I had decided to have the baby in.

I knew that I wanted to use the bath as it had worked so well in my labour with Emily. We decided that it would be best for me to be upstairs when in full labour, as it would probably be a struggle to get down the stairs after getting out of the bath. She asked me to create some space in my bedroom for her to use and we would prepare the room once I was in labour. I packed a bag for the hospital just in case I decided to change my mind.

It was then a case of waiting for the inevitable to happen. I felt very happy with what I had decided. The only thing that preyed on my mind was Emily, my two-year-old daughter. I knew that if I went into labour in the middle of the night I would have to get her out of bed and remove her from the house. I felt that she was just too little to see me in such pain and would get very scared.

My mum asked me a few times if it would not just be easier to go into hospital. If I went into labour in the middle of the night, Emily would not be disturbed: my mum would come to the house and I might even be back from the hospital by the time Emily had woken up. I think my mum could see that it was worrying me and was trying to offer a solution. However, I just knew that I didn't want to go into hospital and that staying at home was the right thing for me to do. I was prepared to move Emily in the middle of the night if I had to.

I went through the motions for the next few weeks. I saw the doctor for a final check up. He said he could see from my notes that I had decided on a home birth. When asked for his opinion, he told me that he would prefer me to do it in the hospital due to the unforeseen risks but he did not try to influence me in any way to change my mind. He just said, "Good luck," and that he hoped it would go well for me.

I had quite a few evenings of feeling strange, then finally the big day arrived. It was Sunday 14 August 2005, the weekend of the Ashes Test between England and Australia at Old Trafford (and two days before my expected date of confinement). I woke up at six o'clock in the morning. I felt strange, a few twinges, so I decided to do the ironing! I knew that if I was in early labour I needed to stay upright to try and get things moving.

Ted and Emily woke up and had their breakfast. We decided by about 9:30am that I wasn't in labour but I phoned my mum anyway. I asked her to take Emily for the day – just in case! I packed for her overnight but expected to see her at the end of the day. When my mum arrived I told her that I wasn't in labour, probably just practice twinges.

I pottered about all morning but by 1pm we decided that I was in labour after all. I was having mild contractions at seven- to ten-minute intervals. I phoned the midwife and she said that it sounded like I was in the early stages; I should keep doing what I was doing and she would speak to me later. I put my TENS machine on and phoned my best friend. I spoke to her for an hour and watched the cricket, pacing up and down my living room, all the time wanting to keep upright.

The contractions were mild to moderate with no real pattern developing. Sometimes they were six minutes apart, then ten, eight and then five minutes. I didn't know if I was coming or going. There was no sign of my waters breaking and I hadn't had a show. I fully expected that the contractions would stop and it would all have been one big 'practice lap'. It was so different from my labour with Emily.

At 4pm my midwife arrived: she wanted to check on me before she made her Sunday dinner! She gave me an examination and found that I was only 2cm dilated and the baby's head was not bearing down fully on my cervix. She told me to call her back when I was contracting every three minutes and if she hadn't heard, she would call back about 9:30. It was demoralising to hear this. All this pain and discomfort and we might not even be halfway there.

Ted and I prepared the bedroom and I had a bath. Within half an hour I was having huge, very painful, contractions three minutes apart. I was pacing in and out of my bedroom with my TENS machine on. I stood and watched the cricket on my portable TV and then with every contraction moved onto the landing and used the banister to hold onto.

We phoned Jackie and she arrived ten minutes later. She gave me another examination and I was only 4cm dilated. I couldn't believe it! The contractions were so strong, lasting minutes at a time. Jackie said to me "if you want to go to hospital, now is the time to go". I told her that I felt confident but couldn't carry on much longer with no pain relief. We decided that I would get into the bath again and then would have some gas and air when I came out. Jackie decided to call the second midwife at this point. Even though I had only been 4cm dilated at examination, she had a feeling things were going to move fast.

Then I had four huge contractions and got into the bath. Within five minutes, I started to feel the urge to push. I had another four huge contractions in the bath, which didn't seem to end. Jackie told me to pant but I couldn't stop pushing. At this point I felt a little scared. The second midwife had not arrived and events were moving *extremely quickly*!

Ted was amazing. We had worked as a team all the way through it. When he left my side I panicked. When he was with me I felt calm, I could cope with the labour. I kept talking to him throughout because by sharing my thoughts and feelings, it helped me to cope with the pain. Labour is so physically powerful and this time it felt immense.

Jackie told Ted, "We need to get Sarah out of the bath *now*" because I had part-delivered in the bath with the membranes still intact. I got out of the bath with Jackie and Ted on either side of me. How I did it, none of us knew but I somehow managed to walk into my bedroom and up onto the bed. Jackie ruptured the membranes with her fingernails and Abigail flew out. She was born at 6:25pm and weighed 7lb 6ozs. I had gone from being 4cm dilated to delivery within 45 minutes!

The second midwife arrived five minutes after delivery and helped to deliver the placenta and membranes. They both decided that I did not need any stitches. My previous scar tissue, from the stitches I had when Emily had been born, had not torn. I was perfectly all right.

I think I was in a state of shock from the speed of delivery. I could hardly talk let alone hold Abigail or feed her. Both Jackie and Kathy were fantastic, staying with us until 8.00pm. There was a little mess, which they cleared up. They made me a cup of tea and put me in the bath. They cleaned Abigail and dressed her for me and settled her into her Moses basket, which was beside me on the bed. I didn't have to think of anything.

Ted managed to start making phone calls and put the dinner on. It all felt extremely relaxed, peaceful and very normal, which helped me to recover from the shock. I was sitting in bed an hour and a half later with a glass of white wine in my hand and a bowl of steaming hot tuna and pasta – delicious! 'Welcome to this wonderful world, little Abigail Elizabeth,' I thought as I gazed at her beside me. I had done it and it had been the most amazing experience of my life. I was so proud of myself for having the strength of character to go through with it.

What motivated me to have a home birth? My previous experience of labour in a hospital had been very good but I was disappointed with the standard of postnatal care. I only felt supported once out of hospital and in the care of the community midwifes. I knew that my body had responded well to labour and I had coped with it very naturally. I wanted to be in my own home and I felt strongly about the normality of it. Women had been doing it for centuries at home, so why couldn't I? Labour didn't scare me: it empowered me. I just knew that I could do it and I *did!*

Nicki's story

Emilia, 2004

I think our desire to have a home birth came out of a general mistrust of the current health system and the influence that drug companies and the suing culture is having on it. We always knew it might not happen and did keep an open mind about it. I have never experienced major pain before and so didn't know if I would be able to handle it and not want to have every drug possible to combat it.

A few weeks prior to my due date the midwife told me the baby was in position and the lump we could quite clearly feel midway up the right hand side of my bump was its bum. For weeks friends and family regularly had a feel of its "bum".

I went about eleven days after my due date and my desire to no longer be carrying a baby round in a really inconvenient and heavy lump grew. My friend is training to be a herbalist so we looked in her books and I made and drank an entire pot of sage leaf tea in a bid to encourage action.

Anyway, I went to bed feeling fine and woke up at 6:30am needing a wee (no surprise there). On the way to the loo I found myself dribbling a bit and then found this didn't stop even after I'd relieved myself. I went back and woke my partner, Stuart, to tell him I couldn't stop weeing myself. "It's okay, Nicki," he assured me, "Come back to bed". I equipped myself with a sanitary pad and took his advice, then fell asleep timing what I thought might be contractions as I had now twigged this might all be baby related. Sometimes I'm a bit slow on the uptake.

It was a contraction that woke me up about an hour later and although I felt quite calm, the feeling of being on a roller-coaster starting its slow and now inevitable ascent kicked in. The contractions continued throughout Sunday but weren't hugely debilitating initially.

The visiting midwife was unsure whether what she could feel trying to get out was a bum or a head and brought in another midwife for a second opinion who assured us it was a head and everything was fine. Early on Sunday evening the first midwife decided that she was still not convinced and sent us off to hospital for a scan to confirm what was going on.

We packed a bag a bit shambolically and set off to City Hospital expecting to return home in a couple of hours time. I was looking forward to having a bath and checking out the hired TENS machine. Although I'd been having contractions all day I had felt a bit in limbo as if labour hadn't really started. The midwife obviously felt uneasy and I had not done a lot of the things I thought I might, such as bathing a lot.

At the hospital I was given gas and air, which was very welcome by then, and a scan which showed a breech baby with the cord wrapped twice and quite tightly around its neck. I was pleasantly surprised to find the staff were all very nice and the consultant treated me with respect rather than coming over as an authoritarian figure. We were left to draw our own conclusions that this was going to be a caesarean birth rather than having the decision pushed on us.

We were then left to wait for a theatre to become available. I was quite upset at first, largely due to disappointment, but also because I wasn't prepared for the speed with which the situation had changed. We seemed to have gone from having a home birth to having an emergency caesarean in a matter of moments once the scan was underway, and making the mental shift was quite hard. However, they left us with the gas and air and taking turns on this cheered us both up considerably. We were actually having fun by the time they came to get us for theatre.

We were in hospital for about four hours in total before we actually went into theatre. The caesarean went fine, although I still find it odd that Stuart has seen my insides. Obviously the birth lacked a lot of the elements we had planned. Rather than having immediate skin to skin contact, I was being sewn up while the baby was carried by an arm and a leg and put under a heater to warm up. They also dressed her in weird things that they had to hand.

When they gave her to Stuart to hold I didn't even dare touch her as my hands were shaking so violently (a reaction to the anaesthetic apparently) and I thought I might damage her. That reads a lot sadder than it actually felt at the time.

I was only in hospital for three days and almost immediately the nature of the birth itself ceased to matter. Obviously being in hospital was hot and noisy, and it just seemed cruel to include Stuart in the visiting hour rules: he had to go home at 8:00 in the evenings leaving me to care for a newborn baby when I'd just been sawn in half and could hardly lift her. But still, the important thing was that we had our baby girl.

Sarah C's story

Luke, 2005

My first son Joseph was born in hospital following a four-hour labour with no pain relief needed and I returned home after one night. As my labour had been so easy we decided to have our next baby at home. Both me and my husband, Phill, had been born at home, and our mums were both very supportive of our decision. However, everyone else that Phill and I spoke to was very negative, possibly because most of them had not experienced an easy labour.

The community midwives were very keen for me to have a home birth, which are popular in the area in which we live. In fact, one of the considerations we had to bear in mind was that they might already be attending another home birth when I went into labour and not be able to deliver my baby.

As Joseph had been born nearly three weeks early the general opinion was that I would more than likely go into labour early this time too. However, this was not the case, and by the time I did go into labour at 40 weeks plus 2 days Phill and I were thoroughly fed up!

I woke at 5am with strong pains, and after three contractions that were five minutes apart Phill woke too. Half an hour later, with my contractions coming every 3-5 minutes, Phill phoned the hospital who got in touch with my midwife. In the meantime I got in the bath, where my waters conveniently broke.

About 45 minutes later, after spending my time either stood up or sat on the edge of the bed, the midwife arrived. My contractions by now were back-to-back and it was a huge relief when I got the green light to push. Fifteen minutes later the head was out and Phill was instructed to lift the baby out with the next contraction, which he was only too keen to do. One more push and Phill lifted our beautiful baby out and announced that we had a son, Luke William. He weighed in at 7lb 1oz.

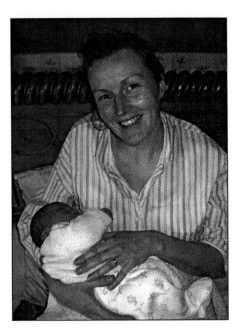

It was only about five minutes later that Joseph came onto the landing looking a little disorientated, but after some reassurance he was happy to sit beside me on the bed. Meanwhile Phill cut the cord and we were all officially a family!

What a textbook labour. It really couldn't have been better!

For another perspective on this experience, you can read Phill's story on p.251

Sue's stories

Jamie, 1992

Eventually the midwife came to me because I didn't turn up for my appointments at the clinic. She surprised me one afternoon – I opened the door and there she was: this tall, middle-aged woman with boyishly short hair, wearing the familiar dark blue uniform. The efficiency of the system was unexpected. It hadn't occurred to me they would send someone out to find me, and then I was worried that I would be in trouble for ignoring the letters. I needn't have been. Barbara was a wonderful woman who treated me with respect and kindness, when I didn't have much of anything like that in my life.

I was just realising what it meant to be living with a compulsive gambler. I hadn't known Michael for that long but had fallen in love completely. We lived in a small ground floor flat opposite an all-night petrol station and next to a coal yard. A wilderness at the back led down to the railway line and a busy road kept constant vigil at the front. I had managed to get the flat through a friend; her dad owned the house and lived upstairs. He took pity on me and let us move in without the usual deposit. I knew the favour was for me and me alone; Michael wasn't really welcome but as the baby's father, and for my sake, he was tolerated.

When Barbara arrived on my doorstep that December afternoon, I had no idea where Michael was. He had gone out to get some milk from the petrol station and had not returned. That was three days earlier. Frantic worry had turned into helpless fury and then quiet despair. I knew he wasn't dead or injured because I'd made all the usual phone calls. He would turn up eventually.

I didn't tell Barbara this, of course. I did my best to look like a healthy, glowing mother-to-be who had just been a bit absent-minded about keeping appointments. She offered to come and see me every week as my pregnancy developed beyond thirty weeks. I gratefully accepted. My one and only visit to the clinic had been an intimidating and embarrassing experience. All the other women and the staff treated me like a teenager, even though I was the grand old age of twenty-two. I was the youngest by a good ten years and decided not to go back for another dose of humiliation.

At some point in the last few weeks of pregnancy I realised that I did not want to go into hospital either. As soon as I knew I was pregnant I had bought a book that explained, week by week, the progress of the developing foetus. I cherished the experience of feeling my body change and knowing what those changes meant. I read everything I could find about pregnancy and devoured the information like a hungry child.

I was, in fact, hungry. Michael returned from his unexplained absences full of apologies and promises. I agreed to take him back. This became a pattern, punctuated by visits to Gamblers Anonymous and GamAnon (the support group for families). I wouldn't have minded so much, except he often disappeared with my money.

I was working part-time as a nanny to four boys, and also qualified for some benefit and free milk tokens. Michael wasn't working. The benefit system meant that payments were made to him. He would cash the giro and then either bin or sell the milk tokens. I hardly ever saw either. For several weeks, I thought we just weren't getting paid and spent hours in the benefits office making complaints. It turned out that Michael made sure he picked up the post before I saw it. I took to sleeping with my purse under my pillow, and when that didn't work, took to hardly sleeping at all.

The lack of money meant that I often couldn't buy food. A huge sack of potatoes was a good investment; I would at least have something to fill me up. Sunday lunch at my dad's was a welcome interruption to the monotony of home-made chips and baked potatoes. My sister worked in a café for a while and would sometimes steal bacon and chocolate bars for me. Luckily I had a craving for rice and brussels sprouts, which could be inexpensively satisfied. I worked until two weeks before I was due and I'm afraid I ate more than my fair share of my charges' after-school snacks.

The decision to have a home birth didn't feel like a big one. Barbara mentioned it as an option and I immediately knew that was what I wanted to do. I'd have to get the agreement of my GP, but she knew her and didn't think she would object even though it was my first pregnancy. A few days later it was all agreed. Michael wasn't happy about it and tried to insist I go into hospital but my mind was made up.

Barbara discussed with me the list of things I would need, which was very short. The midwives would bring plastic sheets and just about everything else. I would give birth in the bedroom, which was bizarrely situated between the kitchen and the living room. All I had to do was phone them when I felt something was happening.

As I got to the last couple of weeks of pregnancy Michael made a bit of an effort to be attentive. He took me to Leeds (or rather, I drove him as he had no licence) to visit his parents. I spent the evening in a smoke-filled room playing Pictionary with his mum and stepdad, sister and her boyfriend. I seemed to be the only one who thought it was weird that his sister's boyfriend was also his step-dad's son. There followed a sleepless night, wondering what counted as incest and whether I could face the four-hour drive home with baby's foot wedged in my rib cage.

The day after we returned from Leeds I decided we had to go and get some baby things. Thanks to my dad, I had already been able to buy a pram. It was my pride and joy: red and gorgeously sumptuous with lots of padding and colourful accessories. I had seen no other like it.

On a wet Thursday in late February, a week before baby was due, Michael and I spent the afternoon shopping. His mum had given me some money as we said our goodbyes, which I stuffed into my enormous bra. She obviously knew not to give it to her son. We bought new babygrows to add to my collection of donated baby clothes. I bought tiny white vests with little ribbons that tied up round the back and packets of muslin squares my mum insisted I would need (and she was right). I had decided to use terry nappies and cleared out Mothercare of all its accessories. I even remembered to buy a cheap camera and some film so I would have photos of my son. For the first time, as we staggered along with our bags, I felt like I was a normal expectant mother.

There was no doubt in my mind that I would have a boy. When I was about three months' pregnant I dreamt I was getting on a bus with a little blonde-haired boy. From then on, I knew I was carrying a son, as certainly as I knew I had two arms and two legs. At the time I couldn't figure out why he was blonde and why we were using a bus; both Michael and I were dark-haired and I hadn't used a bus for years. But my son turned out to be blonde until he was eight or nine years old and Michael sold my car to pay off a gambling debt shortly after Jamie was born.

After our shopping trip we returned to our little flat and I laid out with pride everything I had bought. I was pleased that for once I was ready and organised, a whole week in advance.

At seven o'clock that evening my waters broke. I called the midwife and she said she'd come over soon. To my great disappointment, it was Barbara's night off. Another midwife arrived with a student in tow; she looked uncannily like my dead grandmother but I didn't have time to dwell on that. By nine o'clock everything was happening and Michael was nowhere to be seen. He came back after a while, smelling of alcohol but I barely noticed. I was completely focused on my own body and the amazingly powerful things that were happening to it.

I had prepared some tapes to help me relax and asked Michael to turn on the ghetto blaster in the kitchen. A few moments later I recoiled as Shirley Bassey blasted out 'Do you know the way to San Jose?' It played for a few minutes before my contraction subsided and I had the strength to say that he'd put the wrong tape in and should turn the bloody thing off. I clocked the midwife and my GP exchanging relieved glances.

I didn't need any painkillers. The student midwife tried to put a gas-and-air mask over my face but I fought her off. I wanted to feel everything because it was real and it belonged to me. Even the pain was mine. I wasn't going to allow anyone to take anything from me this time.

Jamie was born just before three o'clock in the morning. I shook uncontrollably for several minutes afterwards and I remember the midwife making me focus on counting Jamie's fingers and toes. I couldn't understand why – I knew he was perfect. I just wanted them to take all their plastic sheets and gloves and leave me alone with my baby. There was some stitching to be done and some other faffing about with my bits, but eventually, they left.

With just the familiar hum of the waking world outside, I could pad softly in my slippers between bathroom, kitchen and bedroom. Everything the same, but different. When tiredness rushed in like a tide and overcame me, I could lie in my own bed, my perfect baby on one side and his father on the other.

Abbi, 1993

February again. Dark days lightened by snow and sliced by cutting winds. I said goodbye to Michael on Jamie's first birthday and began to prepare for another home birth.

I had met Sue at GamAnon. She and I understood each other. She took me under her wing and helped to heal my wounds. We had nothing in common but our gambling partners and, there-fore, everything in common. Our lives were intertwined because our partners became friends too: partners in crime.

So of course it was Sue who would take Michael's place at my side when the time came. She had four children of her own; we didn't miss the irony of her partner taking care of them while she attended the birth of his best friend's child.

June was sunny afternoons snoozing while Jamie slept; sticky nights and swollen ankles; my birthday approaching; other people's holiday plans; nearly time to meet my daughter. Once again, a dream had told me I would have a girl.

Two o'clock in the morning, lying in the dark, I wondered if this was it. Yes, it was. I crept into my son's room. We had moved out of the flat into a little two-up two-down house. It was delightful: a safe and special place. I left Jamie peacefully in his cot and dragged the single mattress out onto the stairs. There was no landing, just a step from the bedroom straight onto the narrow stairway. It was a struggle to bend the mattress round the doorframe, but eventually it gave way and I could slide it down the steps. At the bottom, another tight corner into the living room then one final drag to its position next to the fireplace.

The contractions were quite strong and I was puffing and panting from the exertion, but this was no time to be resting. I realised I was still in the dark, just the orange glow showing through the curtains from the streetlights. I quite liked the privacy and the sense of adventure the darkness provided, so I left the lights off.

There was a lot to do. Towels from the bathroom, plastic sheeting and pillows, tea and coffee to be laid out for Sue and the midwives, a bag packed for Jamie in case he had to be taken out of the way. I would phone Sue and the midwives when everything was ready. As I went through my final checklist, I realised I hadn't had a contraction for a while. Sit down and wait. The faintest of something, perhaps, and then nothing.

I realised I was getting cold. I could just have gone back to bed, but then I would have to clear everything up in the morning and I was wide-awake now. Thank goodness I hadn't phoned Sue for a false alarm in the middle of the night. That might have tested our friendship. Dragging the mattress back upstairs turned into a battle of wills and my swearing nearly woke Jamie up. Finally, everything was back in its place and I clambered into bed and instantly fell fast asleep.

A week later, at 2:30am, I got to do it all over again, this time for real. Sue arrived at about half past three and the midwife a short time later. No Barbara again, but at least it wasn't the one who reminded me of my dead grandmother. Contractions kept me busy as dawn broke. It was soon time to phone my dad to collect Jamie. He took him away, sleepy and still in his pyjamas.

At about 8:30am the phone calls started. My friend, wanting to know if I was going to the mother and baby group that morning. (No, I wouldn't be.) My sister, wanting to know how I was. (I was fine, but giving birth.) The dentist, confirming an appointment. (I would call back, probably.) Someone trying to sell me new windows. (No, I didn't want any bloody windows!)

The living room just about accommodated a mattress on the floor. The best position was in front of the small settee, which was set under the cottage window. As a visitor stood at the front door, they could peer in through the grubby panes. Once the door was open, a tiny porch was all that separated the outside world from me on my mattress.

When the adventure began it was dark, the curtains were drawn and the rest of the world was asleep. Now the whole world was awake and knocking at my door: the milkman wanting payment, my elderly neighbour with a bag of knitted booties, the postman with a parcel, the electricity board to read the meter (he certainly wasn't coming in) and the doctor, followed shortly by an angry lady with a double buggy who couldn't get past the doctor's car abandoned on the pavement. Sue put a notice on the door that said 'Woman giving birth' and we drew the curtains tight.

Abbi was born at about 10:30 that morning. Perfect, healthy, beautiful. No painkillers required. She was put to my breast immediately and we lay there for ages before the midwife insisted she had to take her for a moment. I lay on my mattress and drank tea and ate biscuits with Sue while the midwives cleared up. I never saw a blood-soaked sheet or blanket; Sue took it all away with her and then came back for Abbi's first bath.

Joyce's story

Phillip, 1972

After a trouble-free pregnancy and a ten-hour labour, my first son David was born in hospital on 27 January 1967, weighing 7lb 8oz. We stayed in hospital and went home after two days.

I sailed through my second pregnancy. At that time it was usual to give birth in hospital and I went in at 8:00am after my waters had broken. Richard arrived at 2:00pm on 13 February 1970 weighing 7lb 6oz. We stayed in hospital and again went home after two days.

By 1972, opinions had changed and my GP, relations and neighbours all encouraged me to have a home birth. I attended relaxation classes and met the health visitor and midwife later in my pregnancy. The GP that I had seen for years retired during my pregnancy, so I consulted several doctors.

As David had arrived on his due date and Richard two weeks early, I became impatient when my due date of 18 March passed and we were into April. On my last visit to the GP, I was told I was either carrying a very big baby or twins (there were no scans in those days).

The following morning (5 April) I felt the odd twinge. My husband John went to work and by mid morning I thought I should call the midwife who said she would come later on. By mid afternoon I was getting quite anxious so the boys went to play next door and my neighbour tried to contact the midwife (we didn't have a phone).

John came home at about five o'clock – unable to find the midwife on the way. Eventually she arrived, and by then my waters had broken and I was well into labour. The gas and air equipment proved difficult to operate, but I had already decided by this point that I didn't want any.

At 7:00pm Phillip finally decided to arrive: all 10lb 8oz of him, with a full head of black hair and long fingernails! I was very torn so we were taken into hospital to be checked over. All was well within a few days and we were allowed home. I had to have three salt baths a day for quite some time which was rather difficult with three children!

David and Richard were thrilled to meet their new baby brother, and even with all the delays I didn't regret having a home birth.

Vicky's story

Abigail, 2005

I feel very lucky that throughout my life I have been encouraged to believe that birth is a natural and positive experience. As I grew up, my mother liked to tell us how easy labour and birth was for her and how, after two hospital deliveries, she had a pain-free and very rapid labour when my brother was born at home.

Later in life, as a newly qualified physiotherapist, I found myself working in obstetrics and gynaecology. My three very experienced supervisors instilled in me a belief that a woman's body is capable of delivering a baby without interference. I also learnt of the cascade of interventions that can occur once one medical intervention has been made. I was privileged to observe labour and delivery and found that the whole experience filled me with wonder.

So when I discovered I was pregnant with my first child I felt confident that I could have a straightforward, natural delivery and was keen to have a home birth. My partner, on the other hand, was very nervous about this. When we attended our first antenatal appointment I explained to the midwife that I would like a low-intervention birth, ideally at home, and she was very negative due to this being my first baby. This led my partner to believe that it would be too risky to have a home birth and however much literature I showed him he still remained apprehensive.

As I wanted him to be actively involved with the birth of our baby I felt he needed to be relaxed as well as me so we eventually decided to use the midwife-led unit at the local hospital. In the end I had a very positive birth experience, my son being born after only 90 minutes at the hospital and with the support of two midwives in very relaxing surroundings.

I had not required any pain relief or interventions and the only downside was the long night spent in hospital until we could be discharged home. My partner learnt a lot from this experience so when I discovered I was pregnant again eight months later he was more than happy for us to have a home birth.

We were living in Glasgow at this time and the community midwifery services were run from the hospitals. I chose to book in at the same hospital as before and was disappointed to again be discouraged regarding a home birth. The logic now was that since I had such a positive experience at the midwives unit last time why would I want to risk a different experience at home? What if something went wrong? I left feeling upset but confident that I would get what I wanted eventually as it was only early days.

In the middle of our pregnancy my partner applied for, and got, a job in Nottingham and we were set to move at the point when I would be 34 weeks pregnant. I was sure this would rule out home birth as I had heard stories about needing to book early, but when I called the community midwives they were very positive about me birthing at home and told me all I would need to do was to book in as soon as we moved. And it really was as straightforward as that.

I registered with a GP as soon as we moved and they arranged for the community midwife to visit. She was a wonderful, warm, positive person and filled me with confidence that home was the best place for me to deliver. My only concern was that we were not in our own home at the time. We were staying with my partners' parents. I knew they were happy for me to deliver there and that the odds were that they would be away on holiday as they had a holiday booked for a month around my due date. I was not sure if I would be able to relax if they were there due to fear of disrupting their home.

A week before my due date my future in-laws left for their holiday. I now felt able to prepare for birth; I went out to get plastic sheeting and dug out my old sheets and towels. My closest friend had agreed to come and visit for the week of my due date so that she could take care of my toddler while I was in labour, and seeing her helped to relax me further. I am convinced that my body realised this would be a good time to get things going and labour started during the night on the day before my due date, which was coincidentally my birthday.

I had had a few uncomfortable nights over that last week of pregnancy, so when I went to bed and felt uncomfortable I got up and went to sleep in the spare bed in my toddler's room so as not to disturb my partner, who was working the next day. At around 3am I woke up and thought that contractions might be starting. I dozed for a while then wanted to time them to see if they really were regular and so I got up. The contractions were quite dull and coming every ten minutes and it took me quite a while to decide that I really might be in labour.

By 5am contractions were still quite mild but more regular and I decided food was called for in case things kicked off! After a bit of toast and banana I had a wonderful relaxing bath, enjoying the peace and quiet of a house with everyone else asleep. After my bath the contractions were still quite well spaced but getting stronger so I reckoned that I might as well get my partner up and give him the news that he wouldn't have to go to work. He was very pleased and after initially suggesting I leave him to have a bit more sleep (!) he got up to help me prepare.

I decided to hold off calling the midwife until eight o'clock as I didn't want to wake her. In the meantime I got the room prepared with my plastic sheeting on the floor and sofa and my big birthing ball in the middle. I had thought the lounge would be the best place, as it was most spacious, but then realised that our son would need somewhere to play and decided that my father-in-law's study was the best place; the cosiness seemed what I wanted at the time.

I opened my birthday cards and presents in between contractions and bouncing on the birthing ball. When our toddler woke I was able to help a bit with his breakfast. My friend took over when I felt I really wanted to concentrate more. He seemed very relaxed with her so I felt comfortable taking myself away.

By eight o'clock the contractions were every five minutes. I would describe them as a heavy ache. I was getting through each one by leaning forwards, swaying my hips and focusing on relaxed exhalations. Between contractions I had no pain and enjoyed sitting on the ball chatting to my partner.

I called the midwife who said she would come around in an hour if that was okay to check how I was. I thought that was fine, but by nine o'clock I felt a really strong desire to have a midwife there. She called back and spoke to my partner to say she was stuck in traffic and would be about fifteen minutes. At this point contractions were every 3-4 minutes and getting stronger. That fifteen minutes felt like a long time.

When she arrived she explained that her job was to assist me to birth in the way I wanted and her manner and confidence really helped me to feel strong and in control again. She examined me, to discover that I was 8cm dilated, and called the second midwife to come. I felt so pleased to be that far along and it certainly made the next few contractions much easier.

By now I had decided that I was most comfortable kneeling though contractions while leaning forwards on the ball. I still didn't feel I needed any pain relief and was managing with breathing techniques. When the second midwife arrived shortly after she massaged my back which was lovely.

A student nurse had come with the midwives and was given the job of timing contractions, which were every 2-3 minutes. After a while they spaced out a bit and seemed slightly less strong. I felt very mellow leaning on the ball and would have been quite happy not to move. The lead midwife cannily suggested that I should go to the toilet to provide a sample and get a biscuit on the way.

The thought of a snack got me up and I waddled off to the toilet. On the way I had to step over a barrier we had made to stop my toddler getting up the stairs. This swaying effect seemed to change things immediately and when I got to the toilet I had a really powerful contraction. I felt panicky for a few moments, and very alone, fearing that I would not make it back. I managed a small pee before another really strong and painful contraction and hurried back to the security of the study.

The contractions were now very uncomfortable and long and I felt the beginnings of an urge to push. By the time I got on my knees by the ball I really had to push with contractions and when the midwife looked she could see the head coming down. With the arrival of the desire to push I felt a great let-off in pain and became really excited. My partner was sitting on a chair in front of the ball and I was gripping onto his legs while he rubbed my back.

The midwives guided me fantastically through the next three contractions, enabling me to control the delivery of the head without any tearing. With one more push my daughter was born, still inside her membranes, at 10:47am. While I was turning around to pick her up the midwives covered her so that my partner and I could find out the sex together.

I picked her up and held her to me. Her cord was very short and so my partner was assisted with cutting it. And I was pleased that the placenta was delivered quickly by injection so that I could hold her closer. Within minutes we were all sitting on the sofa, with Abigail snuzzled in my breast taking her first feed.

My friend had taken our toddler out for a walk and when they arrived back everything had been tided up by the midwives and he was able to meet his sister for the first time. Being at home enabled me to give him a hug to help him settle for a nap just like normal. So far we have had no problems of jealousy from our son which may be because it was just like any other day to him.

Giving birth at home was a wonderful experience and as the midwives left at lunchtime we were able to start our lives together immediately with this new member to our family. I am convinced that the feeling more relaxed made for an easier start to breastfeeding, and Abigail herself seemed very relaxed from the beginning. The one downside is that my partner feels that there was too little drama in the whole proceedings – something I am certainly pleased about.

Andrea's story

Stan, 2002

I gave birth to my second son, Stan, at home nearly four years ago. The memories are great, and it still makes me smile with pride that we had one baby at home. I'm lucky because as a midwife I had a great friend, Kerri-Anne, who was prepared to look after me. That was a big reason that I felt confident and safe: I knew who would be coming to our birth.

Kerri-Anne was not in the country when our first son, George, was born, and I did not feel quite confident enough to carry on with the home birthing plans when I went overdue. So knowing my midwife this time was vital to me. I had felt vulnerable before (and I'm a midwife!), so I can really empathise with other women choosing home birth who feel like 'outsiders' or as if they are being 'difficult'. My GP made comments that were narrow-minded and plainly silly, but he just made me feel well informed!

I wanted a home birth so that the environment would be quiet and private, and so that my oxytocin would flow. I wanted somewhere I knew was clean and didn't smell funny. Also somewhere in my motives, I'm sure, was that fact that I've always been a bit different, a rebel!

My partner Phil had got a bit of a shock when George was born. Lots of doctors and midwives rushing around, talking technical and seemingly in a panic. I wanted a more non-medical birth so he could see how it really works.

I started home labour about three days after my due date. And over about 2-3 hours, I spent most of the warming up (latent) phase playing kick-around in the park. I kept it secret for a while as I wanted to make sure that it was really time.

I spent an hour on my own while Phil took George to family and Kerri-Anne (my midwife) was making her way over. I found myself pacing the hallway, leaning against the wall, basically alternating upright positions. I liked my birth ball to sit and roll on. I felt so safe and happy at home alone, so massively relieved not to be getting into a car and going up the A52!

Care arrived as I was beginning to feel a pit panicky: it was all progressing and I knew that I was nearly in transition. I remember Kerri-Anne's strong pressure on my sacral and lower back during contractions really being a lifesaver. Our birthing pool was hurriedly filled. Getting in helped me focus even more and really stay in that place where I could just cope.

Kerri-Anne was sensitive to my need for quiet, being 'just there' along with Phil and another midwife friend. Their words of encouragement were just on the borders of my awareness in those intense moments right at the end!

One word of advice: someone make sure there are film and batteries in the camera that's been put carefully aside for those special shots. We didn't.

Carla's story

Dylan, 2004

Well, I woke on 22 September 2004 (ten days before due date) just before 6.00am, as usual needing to go to the bathroom. When I hopped out of bed I realised my waters were leaking – wow! Not a huge gush, but enough to realise what it was. My husband Joel was just waking and so I gave him the news. "Really," he said.

I had had a show the day before and a meeting with Paulette, our midwife, but it didn't really feel like it was going to happen. Even with the waters breaking the reality of this day actually arriving was hard to believe. I had flashbacks of what Paulette had said to do when the waters break: "Go back to bed if it's in the night; get some rest." So that's what I decided to do, all the time grinning from ear to ear and buzzing on the inside with a mixture of anxiety and excitement.

This being our first baby, and expecting labour to be anywhere from 12 to 24 hours, I told Joel to go off to work and said I would call if anything else happened. So off to work he went. I lay there thinking I might have some breakfast but decided to ring my mum and give her an update instead. That's when I thought I felt my first mild cramp-like feeling, but was not really sure. I finished on the phone and remember timing casually to the next sensation. Ten minutes. Well, I thought, that could be the start of something. Then the next one came seven minutes later, and then a few more and before I knew it they were arriving five minutes apart and I was no longer in bed thinking about breakfast.

Feeling anxious about how fast things were changing, and a little bit worried about being on my own, I decided to give Paulette a call and left her a message. I think it was just after 8.00am. I also rang my dad at some stage, but had started to pay less attention to the actual time and more on the timing. Joel called for an update and I felt sure enough to tell him that he'd better come home. Then I started pacing the house.

It's a bit of fog, but I had a few phone calls from concerned family (funny how quick the news travels). The contractions were more definite now and when I spoke to Paulette they were about 4-5 minutes apart and lasting thirty seconds. She told me it was early labour and she would ring me back about lunch time. Okay, I thought, quite calm that it was still early days.

I paced the house and moving around just felt right. Our two cats stayed nearby the whole labour and seemed calm like they knew what was happening. Joel arrived home just after 10am, although it felt like hours later. By then I knew this was definitely it. It still felt best to keep moving and I was feeling reasonably calm. Things continued to progress and change quite quickly and I really had no sense of time.

We had never done a test run with the pool (something I recommend if you get time) so Joel was busy trying to make sense of the kit pieces, find the watch and time every couple of minutes and run to my side to comfort me through contractions. As you can imagine, it was a fairly stressful situation for him and I was becoming more and more engrossed in labour. The phone kept going too; my mum called back and spoke to Joel to see if I wanted her to come over. All I remember saying is, "I don't know," so she took that as a yes.

I was sick a couple of times but just water since that was all I'd managed to have all morning – I just kept drinking water again, remembering to keep hydrated. I remember Mum arriving, and by which point I had told Joel, who was still struggling with the pool, to forget about the timing and just get the pool up and start filling it.

I continued pacing, with Mum trying to help with the pool puzzle and then rushing to be by my side. I was less and less able to know what to do with myself during contractions and was being quite vocal. The pool eventually got filled and by then I was begging both Mum and Joel to let me hop in – not yet, they said, its too soon. I was starting to feel quite desperate by now: the contractions were intense and I was really starting to feel that I needed the pool *now*.

Joel called Paulette a couple of times to update her: I think he was concerned we were getting really close. I made a couple of comments during contractions about not being able to do this, but Mum and Joel just kept reassuring me and said I was doing great, and so on.

By now it was 12 noon, not that I was aware of the time, and I started to feel a different sensation with each contraction, like my bones were stretching apart. Not long after that I ended up in the toilet feeling the need to bear down. I'm not sure how long I was in there, but I had Mum at my side and Joel coming in and out in between calling Paulette and getting the pool sorted, still not allowing me to get in. Then, thank goodness, Paulette arrived. She came to see me and straight away said, "Lets get you in the pool." Yippee!

I felt really shaky and out of it and remember shivering in the pool. I'm pretty sure it wasn't just the water temperature but a mixture of that and my body dealing with everything. Paulette gave me a first dose of rescue remedy when I got in the pool and that and the relaxing effect of the water seemed to make a huge difference. I felt a calmness come over me and felt really peaceful and relaxed between contractions.

I don't think I spoke a whole lot. Jenny, the second midwife, arrived and I managed to say hello to her. Paulette was checking the baby's heartbeat every now and then, and my mum and Joel were doing trips from the kitchen with hot water to heat up the pool. Time went quite fast; the contractions got closer. A couple of times I asked Paulette, "Please help me," but then they passed and I got to rest again. Paulette got Joel or Mum to pour water down my back during contractions as a distraction, which helped.

Still the reality hadn't set in as to how close I was to having our baby. The pushing stage had started now and it was good to feel I was helping things progress. Feelings of intense pressure and then a burning sensation as the head started to move down. I remember desperately commenting to Paulette after a contraction, "Ahhhh, he's gone back up" – and repeating it, thinking that after all that pushing he was going backwards and I'd have to push him down again. But she reassured me that he would come back down to the same place with the next contraction – thank goodness!

I reached down and touched his head at one stage: it felt warm and had lots of hair. Then, just a couple of contractions later, his head was out. I remember Paulette saying that she could see him and that he was looking around and Mum and Joel came around the side of the pool and could see him too. The next contraction seemed to take forever to come and this was the one I wanted desperately to hurry up.

I started to lift my body out the water as if I was trying to get away from the burning sensation but Paulette told me firmly if I lifted out the water I would have to 'get out' and I didn't like the thought of that so I made a conscious effort to stay in the water. It was five minutes or so before the contraction came that helped me deliver him fully (it felt like forever). All was well, and as he slid out into the water, his daddy had his sleeves rolled up and caught him: born at 1:50pm.

I held him in the pool and put him to my breast like it was the most natural thing in the world and the whole thing seemed so surreal. After twenty minutes Joel cut the cord and had his first real cuddle.

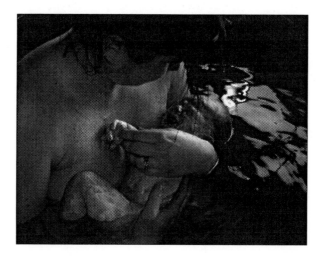

I stood up to get out of the pool and remember commenting on feeling faint then waking lying on my mum on the couch: I had fainted and Paulette, Jenny and Mum had lifted me the small distance to the couch. I was saying, "Where have I been?".

After a bit of a wait I delivered the placenta at about 2:30pm. We then had the first proper breastfeed lying on the couch, and after some pointers from Paulette he went straight on and fed like a champion. Paulette examined him fully and he was a perfect 8lb 4oz, and 52cm long. We named him Dylan.

Joel dressed him for the first time and then he came back to me for more feeding. Paulette showed and explained the placenta to us. In between we made and received quite a few phone calls, and the rest of the afternoon and evening was a celebration with visits and calls from close family and friends, a bottle of Möet and lots of smiles and photos. We had some dinner then went up to bed; Dylan, Joel and I and spent our first night all holding hands and have been sleeping all together ever since.

Our birth was an amazing experience and something that I know we will always remember with pride and joy – the perfect start to an amazing journey. We strongly believe that a home birth is the most natural and positive experience for a family and hope by sharing our story we can encourage parents-to-be to follow that path.

Melissa's stories

Layla, 1998

The main factors influencing my decision for a home birth were that I had been in hospital with my first child and felt that the experience was not natural, and I had not enjoyed it. I had a home birth with my second baby with an NHS midwife. I spent a lot of time in the bath during labour and had my partner and friend there to help me.

I felt at ease with the midwife and my surroundings, and it was close, warm and personal. It was a lovely birth – not traumatic for me or the baby, and we were able to recover in our own surroundings. All my family supported me and my friend was able to be there for me, as at home there's much more space and no restrictions on who can be at the birth.

Tamara, 2002

With my third child's birth the doctors' and nurses' reactions were quite negative as I have a thyroid condition. They often contradicted themselves in the advice they gave me which unnerved me somewhat. This prompted me to look for other options outside NHS care.

In the end we decided to hire a private midwife and a birth pool as I had found water so relaxing and such an aid to pain relief last time. The midwives mainly rubbed my back, took notes, helped deliver the baby and weigh her.

In all my births I used just gas and air. This time I also hired a TENS machine but did not find it useful as my labour was so quick, and I only just had enough time to set up the pool! I just about got in and had my daughter in 4 minutes flat! It was lovely to sink into the warm water and hold her.

Later, I felt cosy and safe in my own bed. It was much quieter than in hospital too! The next day it was nice to have my family around me and the children woke to find a new baby had arrived in the night.

Mary's stories

Egan, 2002

My name is Mary; I am married to Andy. We have two little boys, Egan, aged three and a half and Jay, 20 months. Both our boys were born at home. I am very proud of myself for fulfilling my dream and very fortunate it was all so straightforward. I am sure it would have been a complete nightmare if I had needed to go into hospital.

Although I always said to myself and others that if I needed to go into hospital then of course I would, I was pretty determined that that wasn't going to happen to me! With my second-born it just wasn't even a potential option. I had even more determination it wasn't going to happen to me having heard so many real-life horror stories from friends' experiences of going into hospital. Luckily things were so straightforward that the question didn't even arise.

I was inspired by a close friend of mine, my first close friend to have a baby. You know, when you get to that age when your peers start having babies, it's a bit of a chain reaction with the old hormones! She had a home birth. I remember thinking, well what a wonderful, most natural, common sense thing to do. As with most people, I suppose, I hadn't even thought a home birth was a possibility. Why would I?

Most people only know about births that have happened in hospital. We aren't questioned by anyone, least of all the midwife, as to where we would like the birth to take place. No, I beg your pardon, I *was* asked by my midwife where I would like the birth: Queen's Medical Centre or Nottingham City Hospital! To be fair to her, when I replied, "At home," she was very excited about the prospect, though careful as well not to get my hopes up so early in my pregnancy.

I was very fortunate with the health professionals involved in my pregnancy and birth. I happened to be looked after by a midwife who had had her own children at home and was part of a team of midwives who were very keen to be on call for a possible home birth. It seemed to be the highlight of their year. As for my GP, I don't think I ever saw him or any doctors, so that suited me fine! Not that I'm particularly anti-doctors but the 'medical model' wasn't what I wanted or needed.

So first time around, with Egan, I went all out for a natural home birth. During my pregnancy I was looked after amazingly well by my husband, I ate well, swam, received homeopathy and reflexology treatment, used aromatherapy, went to NCT antenatal classes, and had a very positive attitude about the birth.

When Andy and I look back on Egan's birth, we are filled with amusement by the whole event. It was all rather comical and relaxed. My labour started while I was in the middle of 'nesting': in fact I was making ginger biscuits! An hour or so after the start of labour I rang my husband, who was a student nurse on placement at the time. He promptly came home on the vague suggestion that I might be in labour.

Realising that I didn't have all the right ingredients for my ill-fated biscuits, Andy and I decided to nip to the local shops with the TENS machine attached and working well. I stayed in the car while Andy purchased the necessary ingredients. We were timing the contractions and it was Andy's hope that if he left the car at the end of one contraction he would be back with me for the next. I don't think he managed it! By the time we got back home, ginger biscuits were off the agenda and managing contractions was definitely on the agenda.

Andy contacted the midwife again who we had already informed that labour had started (although they never believe it really has, do they?). When she arrived, she took a look at me and said, "She doesn't look in labour, she's far too rosy" – whatever that means! I was managing the contractions well, which were every 5-10 minutes apart, with assistance from the TENS machine, physio ball, bean bag, aromatherapy and lots of back rubbing. The midwife left with the assurance that she would have time to go home to give her children their tea and be back in plenty of time for the exciting bit as 'first births can be over many hours'. We were fine with that and we carried on as we were.

The contractions slowed down a bit while the midwife was with us: a similar but less drastic effect to what happens to many women when they enter the hospital environment. As soon as she left they sped up with a vengeance. About half an hour after she left I was getting the sensation to push, which anyone who has experienced will know is very difficult to ignore. With Andy's notes from his midwifery placement in hand (only joking) he rang for the midwife to return as quickly as possible. She did so promptly, just twenty minutes before Egan was born.

When she arrived, I think she was a bit taken aback by how advanced in labour I was. My priority was for her to get the gas and air set up and plugged in, thank you. She was trying to do that for me, although her first attempt was quickly flung to one side by me as nothing was actually coming out. She was also trying to get the rest of her kit in, ring the second midwife and put on her gloves to deliver the head which was well on its way.

Seven hours after the first twinge of labour, Egan was born with my husband present and one very surprised midwife. For home birth two midwives should be present; the second one never got there in time for the actual birth, but thankfully came to help clear up the mess!

The midwife and my husband were great. I remember hanging on their every word while I was pushing. It was all very quick and just amazing. I was soon propped up in bed with my beautiful baby boy of 7lb 1oz, chatting away with both midwives while they cleared up around me. How lovely it was to be in my own home with my comforts around me and my own bathroom to have a shower in.

The ginger biscuits were not completed until the next day, but as I said they were doomed from the start. They ended up in a congealed mess at the back of the oven. I can't have placed them properly in the oven: I blame the hormones!

Jay, 2004

My second home birth was much less eventful. It was quicker, taking just five hours from the first twinge, and Jay was bigger at 8lb, which would explain why as a petite woman I needed rather more than the twenty minutes of gas and air provided.

The midwives were very much more on the case this time given my history. I even had two midwives plus my husband! Egan quite naturally spent the last three hours of the labour with his grandma and promptly came home again, once we were all looking respectable, to his new baby brother who had a present for him in the Moses basket. We wouldn't have had it any other way.

The only problem with either of my home births was that we didn't have the right size nappies in the house! But we took advantage of 24-hour supermarket opening. The only real negative aspect for me, with Egan, was that I had real difficulties breastfeeding and didn't have anyone on tap to assist me.

Visiting midwives weren't enough. We got through it, though, with assistance from La Leche League, who were amazing, and I successfully breastfed both my boys for the first year of their lives.

People's responses to my planned home births are quite interesting. They fit into two categories: the supporters and the cynics. People have been very quick to show me which category they fit into. It seems to be a subject that everybody has quite strong opinions about. Supporters on the whole have been my close family and some of my friends. The cynics, strangely, have been some of my closest friends, which has surprised me. Plus, of course, people who have had horrendous hospital births, and others who just have a poor understanding of the positive evidence base for home births.

Comments such as "You're brave" or "I just wouldn't want to put my baby at risk" irritate me. I actually think it would be more brave of me to go into hospital for a birth. And as for risks, I chose to have home births because I wanted to reduce the possibility of having any of the medical interventions which come with their own risks and side effects. And that's exactly what we did. There's not one part of me that would change the unique experiences we shared as a family.

For another perspective on this experience, you can read Andy's story on p.225

Debbie's stories

Jake, 2002

My mum had twelve kids, and eight of us were born at home. Funnily enough, I'm the only one of us that's actually had a home birth, but a lot of my sisters are nurses so they probably just think of all the risks. One of them did have a baby at home but it wasn't planned: the baby just came whilst she was on her way upstairs and her husband had to deliver it! My other sister had wanted a home birth, and a water birth too, but I think she was talked out of it in the end. She didn't even get to use the water in hospital and was a bit disappointed. So I just didn't want to get all worked up when I was pregnant with my first.

I had Eugenia at hospital just because it just seemed it was the thing to do. My sister's a midwife and I talked to her a lot and she encouraged me to have the baby in hospital. She lives in Scotland, and if she could have been near me when I had the baby then I think she'd have felt more able to be involved and help me.

My hospital experience was very positive. I was booked into a low risk unit, and the only hitch came when I called to tell them I was in labour and was told there weren't enough midwives to staff the low risk unit so we'd have to go onto labour suite. But when we arrived the unit turned out to be open after all, so we got to use it in the end, which was great.

It was a large room with a big bath in the middle of the room, we'd brought our own music and there were loads of birth balls and low lighting and the whole effect was very calming and relaxing. We were left in private and really enjoyed it. About half an hour after being assessed and being told I was 2cm dilated my waters broke. We pressed the button to let the midwife know, she ran in and Eugenia was born. Just like that. I remember her saying, "God, you're good at this. We'll see you next year!"

It was the experience afterwards that I didn't like, on the wards. We transferred up in the middle of the night and I was worried about waking other women up. You worry if your baby cries that it'll disturb everyone else, so you don't get any rest. Since she was born at night Jon had to go home. He was self-employed at the time and so was immediately busy with work again. The next day everyone I knew was at work, so I had no visitors and was on my own all day. Jon couldn't get back until six o'clock the next evening and I just wanted to be out of there.

But the birth itself is a really good memory and I honestly wouldn't have been disappointed if I'd had to go into hospital again with the next one.

We were still living in London when I had Jake. I had had such a good pregnancy and such an easy birth with Eugenia that when I was pregnant again, and had the same midwife, she automatically said to me, "So are you going to have the baby at home, then?" And because she was so proactive and just said it to me straight, I said, "Absolutely, yeah, of course I am." It was lovely. Childbirth has never scared me, even the first time. It was never an issue, I just never felt scared. It always seemed something completely natural. If I'd had any problems in any way then maybe I might have worried a bit, but I just seem to get really serene in pregnancy.

Jon, my partner, just said, "All right then," and that of course he'd stand by me 100%. I remember my doctor was really negative though: she kept telling me off every time she saw me. I bumped into her in the swimming pool once and she asked me please not to have him at home, and when she came out to do his postnatal check after he'd been born she said, "Now you're not going to do that again, are you?"

He was five days overdue, and when it started I knew exactly what was happening. You know the signs once you've had one, and you know its not going to stop!

Contractions started about 7:30 and I phoned the hospital, and they told me I'd have to go in after all because there weren't any midwives available to come out. So suddenly I had to start planning and pack a bag and make arrangements for Eugenia. I contacted my childminder who said Eugenia could go and stay with her for the night. She came and picked her up and then suddenly, at nine o'clock, a midwife appeared and said "No, no, you can have the baby at home. We've got somebody now." It was really weird because we were all set up for the home birth, so to be told we had to go into hospital and *then* to have to change back to home again was mad!

They checked me out and discovered I was only 2cm dilated so they told me to call again when I was ready, and then they left. After that we just relaxed and chilled out, and I had a bath. It was really nice. By about eleven o'clock the contractions were starting to come on quite strong and at about half eleven I called the midwife. I'd forgotten I had to give them about half an hour to get there and they finally arrived just after midnight, along with a student midwife, who I'd already agreed could be there to watch. And about 25 minutes later Jake was born.

We were in the bedroom for the birth itself. I used the bath and a TENS machine for pain relief, but I found it easiest being up and about and walking around. I was labouring quite heavily when they arrived and they said it was going to happen very soon. Then my waters broke, and they mentioned it looked a bit green because he'd done a poo in them. I quickly got on the bed (I don't know why – I think because I had quite a small bedroom, and they bring so much equipment, it seemed the best place to be!) and he was out right after that. Jon said he literally just flew out and onto the bed. And we went, "Oh, it's a boy!" Jon was delighted. He cut the cord and Jake went straight to the breast and fed and it was just great. It was so relaxed. I didn't know the midwives who delivered him, we'd never met before but it didn't matter, they were just very efficient and got on with it.

Jon was euphoric, he's always said how lucky he is that I have such easy births, and that I've always been so relaxed. His experiences of birth have been wholly positive. He does say he feels like he hasn't really got a role when I'm in labour, but I tell him he absolutely has because I hang on to him through every contraction.

The midwives cleared up very quickly and went away and we sat there having tea and toast, in our own surroundings. Its so lovely: you don't have to go anywhere; you don't have to worry about your child crying and disturbing other mothers on a ward. And Eugenia didn't arrive home until the next afternoon so we had a lovely time on our own, just the three of us, before the childminder came round to drop her off. She was so excited and utterly made up by having a brother.

Lara, 2005

When we moved to Nottingham and were thinking about Lara's birth I thought there was no way I would consider not having the baby at home. Compared to my doctor in London, my new doctors were very pro home birth. But what was really good about the midwives in our new area was that they arranged for me to meet four or five of the midwives in the team so that hopefully I would know whoever was going to deliver me. Lynn, my named midwife, was lovely.

Eugenia had been 8lb at birth and Jake was 9lb, so Lynn did say that if it looked as though the third was going to be even bigger we might have to discuss the possibility of a hospital birth, and I wouldn't have resisted. Jon was utterly supportive. He was happy to leave 100% of the decision-making to me, though I think its really important to include him in the decisions and for him to be happy with them as well.

There was supposed to be a student attending this birth too, but in the end it was all too fast and we beat her to it. But what was really special was that in the end we had my midwife Lynn at the birth.

My mother-in-law arrived on the Friday night, but I wasn't really expecting things to happen yet and I felt a bit like I'd got her there on false pretences. So I was in denial when contractions did start on the Monday. They weren't really very strong, and with Jake I'd had a few contractions some days before labour actually started so I didn't really think these would come to anything.

They started very mildly at about 11:30, as I was standing in the post office. By one o'clock they were starting to get a bit stronger. We were all due to go to Eugenia's Christmas play at school that afternoon. I had decided that I was still going to go, and had my coat on and was about to leave when Jan, my mother-in-law, said, "You *are* having contractions, aren't you?" When I said yes, and admitted they were coming about one every seven minutes, they decided between the two of them that I should probably stay, and I'm very glad I did!

I had a bath instead, and the contractions actually slowed down a bit and I didn't have one for about fifteen minutes. I didn't think very much was going on so I got out and suddenly they started coming on really strong. By three o'clock they were fast and furious so we called the midwife, which turned out to be Lynn. She got there in twenty minutes and by then they were really quite intense.

When she arrived and had got all her equipment in she could see it was all going to happen soon and asked if I wanted some gas and air, which I thought was a good idea. It had come on so massively once I got out of the bath. I think it must be similar when people get their waters broken: it just really kicked in.

Everything was happening so quickly it was all a bit manic, and there was quite an intensity about it. Lynn suddenly remembered to check the baby's heartbeat, which was fine. Then I heard the kids arriving home with their grandma, and I could hear them running upstairs and I knew they were going to come into the bedroom. As they arrived through the bedroom door I was having a really massive contraction, and I knew that my waters were going to break. I was leaning on Jon for all I was worth, and talking to the children as calmly I could going, "Yes, Mummy's having a bit of pain. It's a bit sore, but everything's okay, and this is gas and air." And then my waters just gushed everywhere: all over the wooden floor, and Jake was suddenly standing in a pool of water!

I suggested Jan might want to take the kids out at this point because I thought 'That's it, the baby's coming.' Lynn had just got off the phone, telling the second midwife that it might be half an hour, it might be two, and not to rush, when I shouted, "I'm going to have the baby. Now!" and launched myself back onto the bed. I was terrified the baby was going to shoot out and land on the floor with a bump! And out she flew, just a couple of pants later. I think we were all quite shell-shocked, because it was *so* fast. We didn't even know what we'd had for about five minutes; neither of us even thought to check. We just accepted that we'd had this baby and it was perfect and that was fine, and then it was like... "So what did we have?"

It was lovely for the kids, because Lara was so nice and clean and they could come in and see that this baby who'd been in my tummy was suddenly a reality for them. In fact, she had the tiniest spot of blood on her head, and Eugenia came over and very maternally just wiped it gently away.

I've asked Eugenia since, "What did you think? Did you get frightened? Did Mummy look like she was in pain? What did you feel?" And she said no, it was lovely, it was really nice. So she wasn't scared or anything. You do worry a bit about how they'll feel, but Jon said I don't make any noise, I'm not a screamer, so there was nothing really to upset them about the experience. It helped that there was no blood or gore or anything like that.

It was such a positive experience for everybody. For me, for Jon, for the kids. I don't see any reason why this shouldn't be a really positive influence on the kids' outlook on their births in the future.

Pamela's stories

Sorcha, 1992

I suppose wanting a home birth was a long time forming in my mind. When I was in my late teens, my older sister was expecting her first baby and wanted a hospital 'Leboyer' birth. I was living with her at the time and went with her to one of her NCT antenatal classes, and I remember it started various ideas going around in my mind.

My sister still says she hadn't been 'brave enough' to give birth at home. She went ahead with her plans for a birth with low lighting and calming music, and it was apparently only at the point when my nephew's head was supposed to be crowning that they realised (what was going on??!!) that it was a breech birth. On went the bright lights, off went the music, and in came a posse of obstetric students to witness a breech delivery. My sister felt violated and, 26 years later, still cries when she talks about it.

Much later, when I was in my late twenties, having just met my husband-to-be and bemused by how broody I felt, I worked for six months on a mother and baby monthly magazine. From reading their letters I got a real insight into women's experiences and feelings about their level of care in hospital.

And so I started reading… One particular book impressed me beyond all others, *Safer Childbirth: A Critical History of Maternity Care* by Marjorie Tew. Apparently, Ms Tew started out wanting to write a book about how much safer it is to give birth in hospital than at home. While researching, again and again she found the statistics showed that indeed the opposite is the case – for the majority of healthy women – and so she went ahead and wrote a very different book!

My husband wasn't very sure about home birth. Not surprising really as his only relatively recent experiences of birth were those of his sister and a close colleague's wife, both of whom had had caesareans. However, I knew I didn't have to fight the point, as at the time of mentioning it I wasn't yet pregnant. The drip-drip effect of my increasing knowledge was a strong influence on him.

At least a year before I conceived, I asked my GP what was the usual thing she said to a patient of hers when first pregnant. Every other word she said seemed to be 'hospital'. So then I ventured: "What are your views on home birth?" She replied "If you want to kill your baby, that's the best way of going about it." Although horrified by her response, and having made a mental note not to see her during my pregnancies, I have since come to recognise and understand this reaction.

In a GP's practice home birth is rare. The GP's obstetric skills are, at best, rusty, and at worst, non-existent. But it's worth remembering that the GP has no legal requirement to attend a home birth in the first place, so their comments on ones choice are totally irrelevant.

And so to my first pregnancy and birth. I'm lucky, I take after my mum who had six children with no major problems. And I had none to speak of either except at the eighth month when I discovered my baby was breech. My midwife had not been happy with my desire to give birth to my first baby at home – it came to light she'd not attended a home birth for years and had worked so long in a Special Care Baby Unit that I think she'd long forgotten what a normal birth was like.

With hindsight I think I should have asked for a different midwife, but she only worked days and I felt certain all babies were born during the night. I went to an acupuncturist to try to turn the baby and spent uncomfortable periods at home on my back with my legs up the stairs. By the onset of labour, baby was head-down.

Quite by chance I had Caroline Flint as my NCT antenatal teacher. She had been a midwife for many years, and still is. She's also a home birth protagonist, author of the book *Sensitive Midwifery* and onetime President of the Royal College of Midwives. It was wonderful, after months of feeling I always had to defend my stand on home birth, to have Caroline actually ask the eight other couples in the class the question the other way around: "Why haven't you chosen to have your baby at home?"

When my consultant browbeat me during an appointment, it was Caroline who put me in touch with AIMS (the Association for Improvement to Maternity Services) and Beverley Beech (its chair) who was so supportive and helpful.

Caroline arranged a post-babies group one evening about a month after the last mum-to-be's due date and in the intervening weeks she suggested we all meet up at each other's houses once a week. I offered to be host the day after my due date of 6 October, saying, "This baby's bound to be late." All my brothers and sisters and I were born after our due date and my menstrual cycle is on the long side so it seemed a safe asssumption.

We all had a very enjoyable evening, and just as the first couples left to return home at about 10pm, I had a show. Once the last couple had gone at about 11pm, my waters broke in a trickle. Although excited, I remembered Caroline's advice: try to get some sleep, which is what we did.

I woke at 5:10am and decided to make the bed up in the room I assumed I would give birth in. I made it normally, then put plastic sheeting over the sheet, then an old sheet with old towels over that, so that once baby and placenta were delivered, just the plastic and soiled sheet had to be taken off to have the bed ready-made below.

It was virtually a textbook first labour: show; waters broke; slow and steady progression of low back pain (6am, 1cm dilated; 1:30pm, 3cm dilated; 5:45pm, 9cm dilated; 6:15pm, fully dilated). The midwife, Pieka, came and went as I wanted her to and as she saw fit, so my partner and I were left together – I was comfortable with this, he a little apprehensive.

I stayed upright throughout, except when in the bath, and was mobile, sometimes pacing, sometimes leaning against a wall just circling my hips which seemed to ease the pain. I ate and drank when I wanted; I didn't have to share the loo with strangers; and familiar sights, sounds and smells all went towards feeling safe and secure.

Contractions seemed to alternate in strength: if one was strong and longer, I knew the next would be less difficult to cope with and shorter. A couple of times I got the shock of experiencing double-peaked contractions: just as the first peak was going, a second came from nowhere!

At the end of the first stage I had what is referred to by some midwives as the 'rest-and-be-thankful' stage: a period of limbo between the opening up contractions pulling the cervix open and the pushing contractions of the second stage which are quite different. This is a time when a woman can regroup and, as long as she's not hurried, can gain a lot of rest and can recharge herself ready for the pushing which is where the word 'labour' comes into its own!

It was during this stage that the second midwife, Mary, arrived. I knew Mary a little from an antenatal visit or two, but it wasn't just good to have her there because I'd met her before: by coincidence her voice was very similar to my mum's best friend's voice. It was a wonderful, reassuring feeling of OK-ness hearing this familiar sound. Something like this is so unexpected, so unplannable, and underlines the belief that there is a profound comfort in familiar sights and sounds which enables labour to progress unhindered.

It was unfortunate, though, that my midwives were a little too busy timing my contractions and were keen to get my labour into the second stage. I think I did a lot of fairly useless and energy-wasting pushing. Having said that, even though they timed the second stage from full dilation, it was still fairly short. Thirty-four minutes: a huge effort but (hard to believe) totally painless.

I gave birth on all fours on the bed. I had tried squatting on the floor leaning on the side of the bed, but my legs couldn't take the strain. I had been urged by Pieka to be on my side with my partner holding my right leg in the air (painful and *very* undignified – although having your ankles up in stirrups for assisted deliveries in hospital is probably far more so!)

It was so strange pushing, as I had no idea when to push – I wasn't feeling any contractions, no pain, just being told to push by my midwives. Then being told *not* to push, enabling the baby's head to be born slowly to prevent tearing my perineum. My daughter was in a hurry, though, and her shoulder tore me slightly. I remember not daring to look down on the bed between my knees. I was still on all fours with a hot, wet mass of life already crying, so small and vulnerable, in the foetal position still connected to me. The umbilical cord was cut once it had stopped pulsing and turned white, and I held my baby in my arms.

I'd decided not to have the injection to assist third stage: from all the reading I'd done, I found it difficult to detect any benefit from having it routinely. Again, I don't think my midwife was happy, but I put our new little baby girl, Sorchia, to my breast and that helped my uterus contract down. Pieka pushed on my abdomen while pulling very gently on the umbilical cord to see if it was ready to separate from the uterine wall.

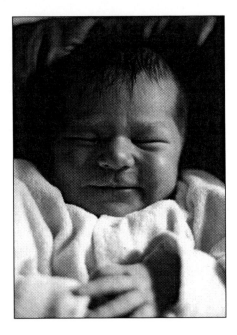

Unfortunately neither midwife wished to be the one to stitch up my tear, so I witnessed a "You can do it"– "No, you can do it" Laurel-and-Hardy type conversation. Eventually Mary stitched me up. The stitches fell out after a couple of days and the wound 'gaped' yet healed beautifully – I had a daily soak in a bath with marigold, garlic and other herbs in a big muslin which turned the bathwater yellow as recommended in Janet Balaskas's book on pregnancy and birth.

The midwives tidied up and once all the checks were done on baby and me I got into bed at about 9pm with a bowl of homemade minestrone which my partner had prepared. Nectar!

Sorcha slept alongside our bed in her Moses basket and woke us the next morning at six. I will always remember the three of us lying in bed, the proud parents flanking their new daughter and gazing adoringly at her. She was perfect. I can't really describe how I felt when I became a mum for the first time. So many emotions, some conflicting: every year has had its joys and challenges. That little baby is now thirteen.

I went on to start a home birth support group within the NCT in the Croydon branch in London where I used to live and ran it for five years, to help other women who may have experienced negative reactions from medical and maternity services. Some of these women had been told downright lies about what they were or weren't 'allowed' to do.

I also trained as a doula (birth attendant) and have supported women and their partners during four births. Now I aim to start midwifery training. My impetus isn't my agenda of birth at home, and certainly not because I'm particularly maternal or love babies: it's more about empowering women during what I believe is one of the most important experiences of their lives.

Alice, 1995

I had had my first baby at home, so one might have expected my second to be straightforward. I guess the pregnancy was, except for a little spotting early on, and the need to have lots of rest – my boss was really putting me under pressure at work, annoyed that I could be so lacking in commitment to my job as to get pregnant a second time and make life in the office so inconvenient.

The due date came and went. My first child had arrived two days after the calculated date, and this baby wasn't going to turn up any other time than when it wanted to. I think I surprised our neighbours, who had no children of their own, when I said I was in no hurry: broken nights aren't my idea of fun! Especially with an older child of nearly three to look after too.

I woke up at 6:20am on the Wednesday with mild period-type pain and rang my oldest friend Alison who'd agreed to be with me. This was very opportune as it turned out, as my partner had been so busy on the building work of our new extension that he got a migraine and wasn't able to be any support. He sought a dark room and slept almost the whole time. I told Alison not to hurry, as it could be some time. She said she'd come after the rush hour. I took my daughter to nursery and let them know that my mum or another friend might well pick her up.

When Alison arrived I was making the beds and vacuuming, having already dusted the house and put some washing in the machine: talk about nesting!

I started timing contractions: only thirty seconds maximum every ten minutes. We played Scrabble. I rang the community midwives' office a lot later and a midwife came out to check me at 4pm – only 1cm dilated. Having filled the pool, which only took an hour, I collected Sorcha from nursery and took her to a friend's house nearby where she had her dinner and played until her dad picked her up at 8pm.

At 6pm I got in the pool for an hour (probably too early as it turned out), then had dinner, and put Sorcha to bed. At 8:45pm, having taken out a few buckets-full of cooled water and topped the pool up with hot, I got back in the pool.

The midwife came out to examine me but at 11pm I was still only 1cm. I was *so* disheartened – I could not believe it. Nancy, the midwife, thought that as I wasn't in established labour (from 3cm dilation on) I might well have slowed things down by getting in the pool too soon. She suggested I rest, stop timing contractions and call her again when they were at least a minute long and no more than five minutes apart. She left at midnight.

My partner was feeling rough with the migraine and felt very low too. I was so glad Alison was there. She slept in the nursery although she said later she found it difficult, as she was so excited. I slept for about 15 minutes and was then woken by a *huge* contraction, which left me shaking and seeing stars when I closed my eyes.

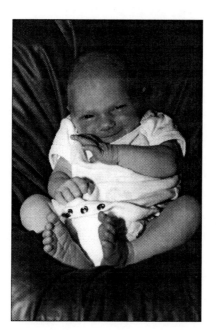

I decided to get out of bed (where my partner was fast asleep!) and sat on the edge of the bed in as floppy and rested a pose as I could. As each contraction came, I stood up, leant over the window sill and blew out. I continued like this in the dark until 2:30am, then went downstairs wondering whether to wake Alison, but didn't. She came down at 3am, and resumed timing. I didn't want to get back in the pool after what Nancy had said so I sat on the edge of the sofa between times and leant against the wall with each contraction, blowing and making sounds.

At one point I was almost sick but managed not to be by swallowing a lot and focusing on my normal breathing. Alison stayed quiet between contractions, followed my lead, and told me the frequency and duration of contractions every 20-30 minutes.

I started to feel very hot and the contractions were ranging from 3-5 minutes apart so we rang the labour ward. At 4:55, Alison answered the phone from Nancy as I was having a contraction and then I threw up, just lots of Lucozade (no dinner!) but a very good sign that things were progressing well!

I was sweating a great deal at this stage, and I was very aware that I stank of onions, due to eating coleslaw earlier, I think. I went upstairs to get Eamonn to ask him to heat up more water for the pool and to tell him I'd called the midwife again. I was still retching, burping and sweating.

At 5:21am Nancy arrived. She felt my belly as I was standing having the next contraction, and then my waters broke: there was fresh meconium staining!! She quickly covered the sofa with absorbent bed pads and told me to lie down; I told her I couldn't and she ordered me to. She rang Josie (another midwife I'd met during my pregnancy who wasn't on call, but who lived closest) and told my partner to get the maternity pack.

I could feel the baby's head coming. I was breathing and blowing like my life depended on it! It was such a weird combination of sensations: burning at skin level, yet from deep within me, an involuntary and uncontrollable swelling expulsion. Nancy told me not to push. I said, "I'm not!" The head was born and the umbilical cord was tight around the baby's neck, so Nancy clamped and cut it, and the baby, another girl, slithered out onto my belly. It was 5:38am.

There was no response from the baby, so Nancy slapped her a bit and used the mucus extractor. I turned her over to allow the mucus to drain naturally. She was fine: she started to breathe and squirm and cry. Her Apgar score was 8 after a minute (-1 for muscle tone and -1 for colour) and 10 after five minutes. I wanted a physiological third stage and had borrowed a birthing stool from the NCT. The placenta just plopped out after about five minutes. No tear this time, only a graze, so no stitches. We hadn't thought of a name for our new baby in advance, yet within fifteen minutes we decided to call her Alice Kate.

We were so proud to go upstairs, and, with her dad holding her, show her to her big sister, Sorcha, who'd slept though all the drama. I'd read that if the older sibling first sees the new baby in mum's arms, there can be greater likelihood of jealousy. This photograph illustrates the absence of the green-eyed monster.

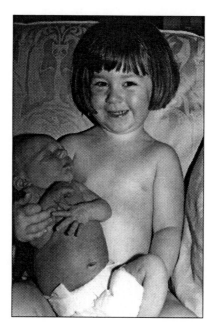

I was told that because of the meconium in the amniotic fluid, we had to be particularly careful: if Alice started coughing or showing any signs of difficulty breathing, we were to take her straight to hospital. Fortunately it didn't come to that. There was a conflict of opinion though – did the cord around her neck cause her stress, which in turn prompted her to have a bowel movement, or should we be grateful for the cord which stopped the meconium getting into her lungs?

Nancy was so apologetic to me for the fact that I hadn't had a water-birth, but I reassured her that my use of water was primarily for pain-relief not specifically for the baby to be born into.

About a week after Alice was born, I talked through the labour with Nancy during one of her post-natal home visits. I asked Nancy what had been going through her mind when my waters broke and she'd seen the fresh meconium. She said that her first priority had been to examine me to see how dilated I was. If I hadn't been fully dilated I'd have had to be transferred to hospital. This is why she told me not to push: as she was trying to examine my cervix, the baby's head was coming down!

Six years later I attended my fourth birth as a doula, yet only my first that ended with a home delivery. They had all been planned home births and I was beginning to wonder whether my two-out-of-two babies at home had been pure luck. I don't know. What I do know is that home birth feels right; having as many or as few friends and loved ones around as you want; doing what you want; eating and drinking what you want, when you want it; the familiarity of everything around you; the unbroken continuity of family life. I can only say that I feel blessed and I'm grateful for everything that brought me to that time and place.

Hannah L's story

Anya, 2003

My partner and I thought about having a home birth as soon as I became pregnant, probably before but I can't remember.

When I was pregnant I remember having conversations with two women about their home births. They were both friends of friends and it was really good to hear these women talking about their positive experiences. One of them was with her husband and he talked about it too – it was really good for Alex to hear how it felt being the supporting partner. We also read some of the pregnancy/birth books and that made us both feel that, ideally, we wanted the birth to be as un-medicalised as possible.

Right from the point when I made the decision to be at home for the birth, I knew that it wasn't something I could assume would happen. It was important to me to be prepared for the possibility of having to go to hospital, and to be prepared for every eventuality, even if that meant a highly medicalised birth or even a caesarean. I didn't want to have the added stress and disappointment of feeling like I'd 'failed' if I didn't have my 'perfect' birth. Having said that, I was certain that I wanted to have a home birth providing everything went well during pregnancy.

My GP was prepared to support my decision and my midwife was enthusiastic and positive throughout my pregnancy and was great at the actual birth. I feel very lucky to have been at a GP's clinic in an area where the community midwives are positive and, I think, experienced in attending home births.

I know from anecdotal evidence and from media reports that plenty of women are actively discouraged, if not refused the option. I don't know what I would have done if I had experienced that. I think as a 'first timer' I would have had a hard time fighting against the medical profession. As it was, of course I had doubts and fears: who doesn't? And I really needed the support and encouragement of my partner and the midwife.

One thing she said to me early on was that I needed a supportive partner who was 100% behind the decision to have a home birth – and I think she is right. On a practical level, I am a big woman and only Alex could have supported my weight when I pushed my baby out. The midwife would have struggled!

Other people's reactions were interesting. Most people said, "You're very brave," or, " I couldn't do it." Most said they would want to have all the medical equipment available for any possible emergency. Interestingly it was more often women who hadn't had a baby who said this kind of thing.

Quite a few of my close friends and family have had pretty difficult births that have ended up in emergency caesarean or forceps delivery. Many of them had felt out of control during the process and had not necessarily been able to make decisions about what was happening to them. It seemed to me and Alex that in many cases the medical profession had at best added to the difficulties and at worst created some of them. I don't doubt that having babies in hospital has reduced the number of women and babies that die in childbirth. However, it is also clear to me that many women do not get the best care they would like during birth.

I think simple things like having your midwife with you throughout the pregnancy and birth can make a huge difference. I had the benefit of a good relationship with my midwife throughout my pregnancy and she was able to assist at the birth.

By twelve days over my due date, I was getting worried that I would be induced and automatically go down the medicalised route.

I had also had a bit of high blood pressure, so that was another possible concern that would land me in hospital. My midwife had already give me one sweep, but now, when she repeated the procedure, she discovered I was already 4 cm dilated.

She assured me I would go into labour later that day, even though I was still going on about being induced, and swapped shifts so that she could attend, which was brilliant. It is things like that which make a big difference to women's experiences: we need a health service that is flexible and responsive to women's needs. I phoned Alex and he came back from work.

I started mild contractions at about 4:30pm, and I think I put the TENS machine on at about 5:30. We had hired a birthing pool which took up most of our dining room and so I spent my labour between the dining room and the sitting room. I spent a lot of time walking around, hanging onto doors and tables during contractions. One of the worst times was when we tried to time the contractions. I stood next to the table and Alex wrote down the times, but I found staying still and concentrating on the contractions made it worse. After that we watched *Thelma and Louise* on TV!

I remember fiercely clutching whatever was at hand during contractions – sofa arms, Alex's hand, door knobs, etc. Quite quickly I got into the rhythm of tensing my hands but trying to relax the rest of my body and breathe deeply. This is something I learnt many years ago as a teenager when I used to get excruciatingly painful period pains and my mum taught me how to cope with the pain. I think the ability to breathe and relax was key to me getting through the labour and although I hadn't done any specific preparation for the birth, I do yoga and this really helped me to cope.

I think the film ended around midnight and the contractions had got gradually stronger and stronger. Alex had spoken to the midwife before but now we rang her again and asked her to come. Alex had filled the pool and I got in at about 1:00am. Immediately the sensation of warmth and weightlessness gave me relief – it felt great being in the water. But then a split second later the contractions got much stronger. It took me by surprise, but quite quickly I got into a rhythm of riding the contractions and then completely relaxing with my eyes closed in-between.

I did worry that my baby was going to arrive before the midwife but luckily that didn't happen. She was able to examine me without too much difficulty. I had my arms over the rim of the pool and I would sit on a stool and stick my feet up over the pool rim and raise my hips so she had access.

Although I had thought that I would want gas and air during labour it didn't really occur to me that I needed it. I was just so focused on riding out the contractions and then completely relaxing and emptying my mind and body in between. Things went on like this for at least an hour, possible more. I remember it being really important that Alex was physically near me. He was rubbing my shoulders constantly with the odd break to make tea and muffins for the midwifes. I didn't like losing the contact and was always relieved to feel his hands touching me again.

I had absolute confidence in the midwife and that made me feel secure. Sometimes my loud, long and deep 'arrrrrrrrhhhs' during contractions would turn into high and shrieky 'ahhhhhs', the kind of noise you make when you're in pain and panicking! At these moments the midwife would encourage me to relax and breathe and helped steer me back to the more controlled state that I had been in.

At some point, probably around 3am, I moved into the transition phase and everything seemed different. The midwife tried to get me to push but at first I was confused and thought I just needed to poo. I had read about it feeling like this but it still seemed like this was a problem. After a while, I remember thinking, 'What do you mean I need to push? What do you bloody think I've been doing?!'

It dawned on me that I actually wasn't pushing but practically the opposite – I was 'riding' the contractions and holding on. I think this relates to the fear that you need to poo and, more to the point, the fear about what happens when you do push – 'Am I going to split in two?' There was a moment when I doubted that I could do it and I remember thinking, 'Right, I'll have to go to hospital and have a caesarean' – but I don't think I actually voiced any of this.

What surprised me was how 'with it' I was: it felt almost like the contractions had eased off. Here I was in the middle of my dining room and I realised that I just had to damn well push with all my brute force! I was finding it difficult to push in the water because it didn't seem to be working and I felt I needed gravity. I also found myself getting cramp in my knees when I tried going on all fours. At this point I decided to get out of the water.

Again, I couldn't go on all fours because I got cramp so I ended up standing, legs bent, facing my partner with my arms round his neck. Each time I pushed I hung from Alex and bore down on him with all my weight. God knows how long this whole period took – I was not aware of time but it didn't seem that long. I remember Anya's head coming out and what an amazing and weird feeling that was. And I remember the brief thought of 'Bloody hell: how will her shoulders and body get out?' The midwife asked if I wanted to touch her head, but I didn't: I just wanted my baby to be out and to be safe and sound. And out she slithered with the midwife catching her. It was 4:45am.

Oh my, what a moment. I think the midwife dipped her in the pool to clean her off – she certainly wasn't at all mucky when she was placed on my chest. But that might have been because my waters didn't actually break until right at the end of labour, and then only because the midwife broke them. Oh wow, that feeling of pure unbridled joy at seeing my baby there, our daughter, and holding her to me. The most wonderful moment of my whole life for sure.

I did get her to latch on to a nipple for a bit but not for long. She was peaceful and quiet and beautiful. There followed a mild panic in which I was losing a fair amount of blood and it took the midwife a while to locate and deal with the source (a few tears in the vagina). I honestly didn't care. I had some gas and air and I just lay there legs akimbo and stared at my daughter who was at this point with Alex. I think it was more scary for Alex who could see all the blood around me on the mattress I was lying on. Eventually that was sorted out and everyone was content.

We all had some tea and snacks and then by about 7am Alex and I were upstairs in our bed and the midwife helped me get started with breastfeeding. We were both totally elated by the whole experience and in awe of this precious little creature. And then we had a giggle thinking 'Right, how on earth do we care for her from now on?!'

And now Anya is two years old and still a joy to look at and be around. We worked out how to look after her, the same way all parents have to – I guess you could call it learning on the job.

Sarah E's story

Henry, 2004

I knew as soon as my second pregnancy was confirmed that I wanted a home birth. I had planned to have a home birth with my first child, Thomas, but an earlier-than-expected appearance changed all that. In total my labour with Thomas had taken three and a half hours so, unfortunately, my husband, Tony, had missed seeing his first child born.

My midwife was fantastically supportive about a home birth. Thomas had been a low birth weight and this meant I had to be monitored more thoroughly during my second pregnancy, but as long as the baby was growing well then the consultant was also content for a home birth to take place. At my 28-week scan it was confirmed that the baby was a good weight (and boy, could I tell as well!) and the planning could begin in earnest.

We set up our spare room for the birth. I had a bed-settee complete with old duvet and plastic sheets if I chose to lie down. I had bought a birthing ball for the first pregnancy which I intended to get some use from, and I had a portable stereo complete with soothing music.

I knew that labour number two was going to be quick and, rather than a trip to hospital in an ambulance being told not to push like the first time, I wanted to feel relaxed and in control. My midwife was very helpful in calming my concerns about the baby arriving before the midwife did and even ran through what to do if that happened.

Two weeks before my due date I was woken at 6:45am by a sharp pain in my lower back, and at precisely the same moment

Thomas woke up in his room and called out. I thought Tony had poked me to get up and see to him. I leaped out of bed and the waters trickling down my leg made it clear that today was the day.

We phoned the midwife immediately and I was rather put out when Tony was told that they wouldn't come out until the labour pains started. He made it quite clear that once they started things would move quickly and they agreed to call back in an hour. I wasn't happy about this but lay back down on my side, in our bed, listening to the Chris Moyles breakfast show. The labour pains started about half an hour later. Fortunately the midwife had obviously realised that we were panicky about an early appearance and she phoned back about ten minutes after the pains started and agreed to come out and check me.

The pains weren't too bad so I just lay in bed while Tony got Thomas up and dressed. Once the midwife arrived Tony felt happy about leaving me to take Thomas to nursery. The midwife checked how I was doing – regular pains, not too severe – and we agreed that as soon as my husband returned she would see how dilated I was.

At 8:30am I was told I was 4cm dilated so I decided it was time to get up off the bed and take a more active role in getting things moving. I went into our spare room and leaned over the birthing ball. The contractions became much stronger as soon as I was upright and in the space of about ten minutes they became really intense.

I decided to move to the sofa bed and lay on my side, breathing through the contractions. Tony held my hand and pressed a cold flannel to my forehead. I didn't look into his eyes. I knew that seeing me in pain must be distressing for him and I didn't want to see that. The urge to push hit me hard and the midwife told me to go with it. I pushed and the baby's head arrived – he was screaming and I could still feel him kicking me inside. We had asked that Tony be the one who told me the sex of the child. I couldn't look at him but I can still remember hearing his voice, cracking with emotion, saying, "It's a boy." We had really hoped we would have another boy.

Tony cut the cord and Henry George was passed to me. He wasn't interested in feeding so Tony held him while I tried to go through a natural third stage (I had had one in hospital with Thomas). This time I had to have the injection but it meant Tony was able to spend time with his second son.

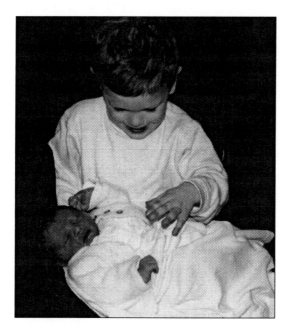

My records show that my first urge to push was at 8.55am and that Henry was born at 9:10am. In total the first two stages of labour had taken less than two and a half hours. The second midwife turned up at 9:30am. I hadn't even thought about pain relief.

I got cleaned up, Tony held Henry, and the midwives left us together. It was peaceful and we were comfortable at home. There was no urgency to do anything. We knew we had a little time before Thomas needed to be collected and we just held Henry and cuddled.

In hindsight I'm glad Thomas wasn't at the birth. I was able to make a lot of noise and that would have frightened him. We had explained to him that baby was on the way when Tony took him to nursery and when he arrived home he was introduced to his new brother. I'm not sure he was that impressed.

We asked people to leave us alone for the first few days although this seemed beyond their control! But we were quite strict when they came, asking them not to stay too long – there is a danger that as you are at home they'll think they're all right to stay for ever.

I can't remember anyone in the immediate family ever questioning our decision for a home birth. Most of the time these questions were from outsiders and they always asked, "What will you do if something goes wrong?" My opinion is that the midwives are the experts but you also know your own body. I had almost primitive feelings to lie down or stand up: my body knew what to do and I listened. I accepted the responsibility that something might go wrong but never anticipated that it would.

I felt calmer in my own surroundings than I ever could in the hospital. You know that you are going to get the midwife's complete attention. And the difference after the birth: well, you get some sleep, which is almost impossible in hospital.

Would I recommend a home birth? Most definitely – there is no comparison.

Pam's story

Sarah, 1971

I gave birth to our first baby, Paul, in hospital on 14 June 1969 and spent five days in hospital. Apart from suffering from mastitis I had an easy birth (six hours in hospital prior to the birth) and decided that next time I would prefer a home birth.

Sarah was born on 23 July 1971 and I wouldn't have changed a thing! The local GP and midwife carried out my antenatal care. A few weeks before I was due the doctor 'turned' her as she was in the breech position. Big brother Paul, who was with me for the appointment, helped the doctor carry out the procedure.

I started labour at 6:30pm while out for a walk with my husband, Geoff, and Paul. We made our way home, bathed and bedded Paul and started to watch *The Virginian* on the television. When my contractions were coming about every five minutes we rang the midwife. She came out and ordered me to bed. (We missed the end of *The Virginian* – there were no videos then!) Geoff was given the job of working out how to operate the new gas and air equipment, and failed miserably!

Shortly after the midwife's arrival my waters broke and during one of my big pushes I passed some 'sheep droppings'! Just before her birth I had some assistance given by a pair of scissors to prevent me tearing too much and almost immediately after that Sarah was born at 9:45pm, at 8lb 4oz, with Geoff cutting the cord. Once it was established that baby and myself were both fine they finally got the gas and air to work! Shortly afterwards the doctor came to stitch me and as he had no local anaesthetic with him I actually got to use the gas and air in the end.

The midwife left us at around 11pm and, with Sarah tucked up in her cot, Geoff and I went to bed. The next morning Paul came into our bedroom and there was great excitement when he saw his little sister and he ran about shouting, "Baby come."

The midwife returned at about 10am the next day suggesting that our dog should meet the new member of our family and we should let him lick her. After lunch that day I got up and started supervising the running of the house again and both sets of grandparents visited to see the lovely new addition to our family.

Although home births were not popular at the time I did not get any resistance from the medical profession. Family, neighbours and friends thought we were very brave and were more concerned than we were that "Things might go wrong". But for me, having a baby is the most natural thing in the world and what better place to give birth than in your own home with a loving husband at your side?

We have all lived happily ever after and our baby girl has just experienced a similar situation with her second baby. The only difference nowadays is that far more information on the pregnancy and birth seems to be provided, which I feel is not always a good thing!

Tracii's story

Tommy, 2005

Home birth was briefly mentioned at my booking-in appointment when I was about eight weeks pregnant. It wasn't a scenario I'd considered or thought practical at that time. What woman would choose to ruin her furniture and flooring? To be honest it wasn't really presented as an option, and I knew so little about it that I didn't really give it a second thought. Instead I immersed myself in more pressing matters.

This wasn't going to be my first experience of childbirth; in fact there are almost eight years between my sons. My elder son was born after a long drawn-out labour lasting more than seventy hours, spent in a now-closed Victorian women's hospital. It was a Bank Holiday weekend in intense heat, with no air conditioning and windows that had been painted shut. The midwives on the whole were pleasant enough, but this was a conveyor belt, and I was not an individual. It was stressful, clinical and pretty unpleasant but, to be honest, I had no idea how deeply this experience had affected me until the birth of my second son was nearing.

I had been putting off packing my bag for hospital, but I hadn't really given much thought as to why this was. Then I had a chance discussion at nearly 34 weeks pregnant with one of my oldest friends, who had recently had her first child, and the subject of childbirth came up. I realised I was really worried about going into hospital: the whole scenario made me feel uncomfortable and stressed for so many reasons. The more we discussed home birth, the more comfortable I felt. No-one had discussed it with me before, and all of a sudden something felt right.

I went home to research all I could digest about home births and decided that at my next midwife appointment I would discuss this option. And so I did. I apologised because I felt I had probably left things a little late to make arrangements, but I was sure this was what I wanted. I wasn't expecting the reaction I got.

First I was told as politely as possible that my BMI (body mass index) had been too high when I had fallen pregnant. Apparently this was one of the criteria for home birth in my local area. I told the midwife that I had been even larger when I had my first son, and that fat or not this baby was coming out.

It's a bit disheartening to be told that you are too large for a home birth, so I pressed my midwife further as to why. I was told she was just following local authority guidelines, due to larger ladies (I'm hardly Dawn French!) having increased risks during labour. I pressed further... what risks? I was informed that I had an increased risk of shoulder dystocia, which is basically where the baby's shoulder gets stuck on the mothers pelvic bone and can be a potentially fatal complication for the baby.

I asked her what studies there were about this. What were the chances of this happening in a smaller mother? And by how much did this risk increase due to my size? She couldn't tell me. On that basis, I said I would do more research myself into the possible risks presented to my unborn baby by me having the sort of figure that meant size 18 jeans had to have a lycra content.

So I researched, and researched, and researched (thank God for the internet!). I found no empirical evidence to support the local health authority's stance on my BMI being a greater risk to myself or the baby should I opt for a home birth. In fact I found little evidence at all: unless I had been seriously obese, the risks appeared to be no greater if I were a size 8 or a size 18. I spoke again to the midwife. I explained that I was fully aware of any potential risks, however remote, and that I still wished to have a home birth.

Then I was told that my routine blood test results had shown my iron level was slightly below the local authority 'guide' range for home births. The actual reading was not drastically low, but just nought point something below the midwife's guide range. I offered to take iron supplements (despite the horrid side effects: black poo and constipation), and insisted that a home birth was still my preferred choice.

I was told more times than I care to mention over the next few weeks that, even though I was only five minutes away from the local hospital, if something should go wrong there would be an increased risk of harm to my baby and also myself. Scenarios ranged from the baby getting stuck and potentially getting starved of oxygen, to bleeding to death due to 'anaemia' and so on and so on.

I had to speak to two registrars at the local hospital, both of whom tutted at me. I could understand if their attitude was based on me making uninformed, dangerous decisions or wishing to harm my baby, but I had all the information, which was more than they had. When I asked questions, the answers were vague, but none of my questions were vague: they were precise and informed. I felt the doctors were not familiar with the whole concept of home birth, and was told directly by one that babies should be born in hospitals. The whole thing had been turned into a battle for me. I really didn't need the added stress of all this at this stage in my pregnancy.

I also have multiple sclerosis, which hadn't affected my pregnancy at all; in fact I'd been pretty well throughout. I assumed that this would be used as an excuse at some point over the weeks, but luckily (probably due to some disability discrimination legislation) it was never raised as a concern. And so it shouldn't have been. To be honest, anyone who knows anything about the condition knows it affects people in different ways. To look at me you wouldn't know there was a problem – there's no wheelchair or walking aids, so of course it shouldn't have been an issue. The way I saw it, I had got the baby in there and I would get it out!

My husband and I discussed the situation lots, and despite his reservations (he would have felt more comfortable with a hospital birth), he said he backed me 100% if the choice made me feel more comfortable. He looked at all the information himself, and knew I was making a clear, informed choice, and that I wouldn't do anything to jeopardise the baby or myself, and on this basis he supported me.

I think because I had researched so much on home births, and could hold my own in discussions with the doctors and midwives, the head of midwifery at the local hospital agreed that the community midwife team would support my choice (then again, I believe they have to by law anyway, although I could be wrong). However, this was on the basis that the very small community team were available. Should one of the other ladies awaiting home birth go into labour before me then I would have to go to the hospital.

It was a possibility I'm sure, but what were the chances really? I believe there were only three others due in the whole of February. Four women, one month, different due dates, going into labour at exactly the same time? I agreed that if this happened I would go to the hospital. I also agreed that if the attending midwife felt that we needed to go to the hospital then I would go. I needed them to see I was not being reckless, that I was only trying to achieve the best situation for me and my baby.

With everything agreed, I had the birth pack delivered and bought tarpaulin, just in case. All I needed to do now was wait.

And wait…

…and wait…

I had tried rasberry leaf tea last pregnancy and wasn't going to try that again; I tried sex, but that was just plain uncomfy; had curries, but just got indigestion; and ate fresh pineapples until I got mouth ulcers. I asked the midwife if she would perform a cervical sweep, but she told me that this was seen as intervention, and as I wanted a home birth she couldn't intervene! *Bugger.*

Two days after the dreaded due date, and my induction appointment at the hospital was looming. I wouldn't advise what I did, but it apparently worked – I got on the internet, and looked up how to perform a 'sweep', which I did on myself. Things got started the following day.

The pain was there, but not regular. My waters didn't break, but things were definitely starting. It was uncomfortable, but I just got on with the day.

I went to bed that evening, but things were too uncomfortable and I couldn't sleep so I got up. Thank God for Sky TV! I watched a great documentary about transsexuals at 4am whilst sitting on my gym ball (by the way, don't bother with an expensive birthing ball: I got mine from Tesco for six quid and it worked just as well!). I didn't want to call the midwife out until I was sure I was in labour. With all the trouble I'd had trying to get a home birth, I didn't want to call them out in the early hours for a false alarm. So I watched TV, rocked on my ball, did the washing up and a bit of tidying, and timed the pains.

As it approached si o'clock I woke my hubby, then rang the midwife to tell her I thought I was in labour and how far apart the pains were (about 4-5 minutes or so at this point I think). She asked me if I thought I was anywhere near giving birth, I told her I had no idea – I'm hardly an old hand at it!

The midwife, Liz, was there within half an hour. She was lovely. I'd only met her once before when I'd had my booking-in appointment months and months before and she had been covering holiday leave for my practice midwife. It seemed sort of apt that it was her for the final appointment too.

Liz examined me and told me that I was 8-9cm dilated, and that I'd done most of the hard work without her. I wasn't sure how long this would take, but I was expecting that the baby would be there before lunchtime. I had bought an enema from the chemists (I really don't like the idea of have a poo at the same time as having a baby), and asked when I should use it. Liz said that now was as good a time as any, so I went to the bathroom. The enema worked and my waters broke too!

At about 7am, my mum arrived to take my eight-year-old son to her house. He was half asleep when he left, and to be honest if I'd known how quick things were going to be I wouldn't have woken him at all! He had said he didn't want to be involved in the birth: although he was looking forward to meeting his brother, he'd seen too much already on the Discovery channel!

Around the same time, the second midwife, Gill, turned up. Liz had already called for her to attend as she didn't have any Entonox (gas and air) with her. I had never had gas and air before and it was quite nice, it really took the edge off the pain and gave me a light-headed feeling.

Throughout this activity my hubby had busied himself getting a wet flannel, not that I was hot or sweating, I think it just made him feel more useful! Through the haze of the Entonox I remember seeing the smile on his face which he was trying to hold just to make me feel better; meanwhile his eyes oozed abject terror, like a rabbit in the headlights!

As the pain increased, I kept thinking that there was no way I could cope with this for hours. Liz examined me and told me not to push yet as I wasn't fully dilated. So I held on through the pain until an overwhelming urge to push came… I did, and with that I heard one of the midwifes telling me to pant as the head was there! I'd been expecting a long haul on this; I'd only pushed once, the midwife had only arrived at my house about an hour before, and the second one had been there about half an hour. This was too easy… okay, not easy, but too perfect! I was pretty shocked at how quickly it all happened.

I panted, and within the next sixty seconds I pushed once more and had my little boy. It was the most amazing experience ever. It was my second birth experience, but this was just too good. It was natural, it was comfortable, it felt right.

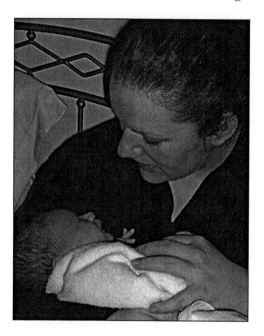

My 9lb 12½oz son Thomas was born at 7:37am, in the same bed he was conceived in, to the sound of Chris Moyles, the saviour of Radio One! There were no horror stories, no tears, no abnormal blood loss, nothing bad. It was all perfect.

I never imagined it would be that fantastic, that life-affirming to be honest. It sounds all floaty and tree-huggy, doesn't it? But believe me I'm not at all like that. If my first birth experience had been like this, I might have had a whole brood!

The midwives cleaned up; there was virtually no mess. They were gone by 8:30am. I was up having a cup of tea in my own home and speaking to friends within five minutes of his birth. Unlike a hospital where you have to do things by their rules and schedules, my family were able to come straight round and see the new addition. I could use my own toilet, make my own tea and toast. These may seem like little things, but it's the little things in life that make us comfortable, and put us at ease.

If a woman is confident enough, and medically able to do so, I personally believe a home birth is the most natural and beautiful start to a baby's life.

Ness's story

Alex, 2005

From the start I had concerns about the birth. It might seem premature to be worrying about going to hospital for the birth at five weeks pregnant, but that was me. I just had an issue with all the rules and restrictions and everyone else's agendas, and I was worried I would end up voiceless. I wanted to be in control, (oh the irony!) but more than that I wanted to look back on a positive experience with no regrets. I had an innate sense that my body knew how to do this birthing thing. After all, it was growing a baby and making me feel sick if I ate the wrong foods and changing my shape from day one: I had to believe it knew what it was doing.

Eventually I broached the home birth subject with my husband, Loz. Initially he sounded cautious: he was already wary of the whole birth thing, wondering whether he would let me down, or pass out at the sight of blood. And I think he still needed to build up a picture of what a home birth would look like.

We had our first midwife appointment at ten weeks, but didn't raise the home birth issue as we were too busy, as first-time parents, trying to understand scans, tests and why pregnancies are forty weeks long.

Working full-time and not knowing anyone else who was pregnant, I took to reading everything possible to find out more about birthing options. As I read I became more and more convinced that I wanted to create a safe, peaceful birth. For many people pain control is at the top of their list of priorities (and I'm not knocking that) but for me I wanted to feel safe, to be in an environment where I didn't feel I had to 'fight' anyone, or protect myself, and I could just listen to my body and work with it.

When I started mentioning that we wanted a home birth to friends and family, there were a lot of comments about being selfish, the risk to the baby, the lack of pain relief – "Was I mad?" Each one of these comments hit a chord and I thought long and hard about them all. I went through stages of feeling sad and angry, as well as scared, that people thought I would take risks with my child, that this was me trying to make a point, or that I was somehow naïve about the pain.

But Loz and I came back to the opinion that the more relaxed our environment was for us, the happier and more comfortable we would be, which had to be better for the birthing experience and our baby. At our next midwife appointment we asked how we would go about arranging a home birth, and she said she would be happy to discuss it with us at 37 weeks, providing everything was going well, my blood pressure was okay, the baby was in the right position, etc.

By this time we were pretty convinced that we wanted a home birth and started to look at alternative pain relief. NHS antenatal classes weren't available to us until week 36, which was way too late for us: we wanted information now. So we decided to go to hypnobirthing classes, which were really helpful. They gave us the chance to explore birthing options and the type of birth we wanted, as well as teaching us breathing, visualisation and the power of positive thinking. All techniques we subsequently used successfully.

Around the same time, we joined the NCT, and contacted a local home birth support group. We were invited along to a meeting, where we explored home births, planned and actual, which was incredibly helpful for us. We needed to hear some real stories, that we weren't the only people considering this, and we benefited from meeting some lovely people. We also came away determined to have a birthing pool, and subsequently bought a birth-pool-in-a-box by mail order.

Our due date finally arrived and passed with no excitement. The next day we went to see our osteopath. She offered to move things along, and by 10:30 the same morning I had the first contraction. We thought we were going to bed that night, but as it turned out, the contractions became too strong, so we spent the night in front of countless episodes of The West Wing.

I used a TENS machine, to some effect, and some Shiatsu acupressure points which Loz pressed during the worst contractions were hugely helpful. But the breathing techniques were the most helpful.

Next morning at eight o'clock Loz called our midwife, Julie, and when she came out and checked me she told me I was 5cm dilated. She had to go and collect equipment but was back for the duration by 10:30 that morning. Julie was excellent from start to finish: supportive but unobtrusive; allowing Loz and I to shape our experience.

Loz started to fill the pool around noon, and it took an hour and a half. Julie had warned us about not getting in too early, so I duly waited for the right moment. I can count on one hand the moments in my life when things have felt as good as when I finally got into that pool.

Unfortunately my contractions started to drop off, so after much walking up and down our stairs to bring them on stronger, and two hours of pushing, Julie advised us that we needed to go to hospital to have the baby. I was hugely disappointed but I knew I had given the experience everything I could, and as it turned out our little man was sideways on, and was unlikely to have made it out at home.

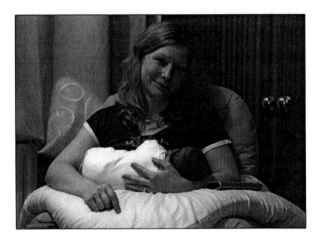

Loz tells the story of the hospital better than I do. Julie accompanied us there and handed us over. As soon as we arrived, decisions started to be taken for us, but to be fair this was no longer a planned situation and we were now looking to the staff for help. Baby Alexander Isaac Glew was delivered by Neville Barnes forceps. No epidural, just Entonox, breathing, TENS, a birthing pool and Shiatsu! The hospital team were lovely, the midwife in charge of us even coming back to congratulate us and give us a hug at the end of her shift.

I did go through a short period of feeling that I had failed – after all, I didn't get to fulfil my vision of handing Alex over to Loz in the birthing pool at home and seeing his face – but we do have a beautiful healthy baby boy. In my mind, we achieved our birth plan. Okay, so Alex didn't want to arrive at home, but the 19 hours of labour at home was, well, great, and I wouldn't change a thing.

For another perspective on this experience, you can read Loz's story on p.227

Rachel's stories

Alex, 2000

Alex was born on Christmas Day 2000 in hospital. Frank was born on 9 February 2003 in a birthing pool, in our kitchen at home. They were the most challenging, joyful and exciting times of my life.

Previous to Alex I had had two miscarriages, which left my partner, Paul, and myself nervous about choosing a home birth. I think in hindsight without my miscarriages I would have had no doubt that a natural home birth was for us. Paul needed the confidence of doing it in hospital first and I wanted the reassurance that if anything went wrong we had all the technology and medical support we needed. I wanted to protect this third baby. Our parents were definitely reassured by our decision of a hospital birth. However somewhere deep down I still fantasised about a home birth.

I loved being pregnant with Alex. He was such a wanted child as you might imagine, and I really enjoyed putting a lot of energy into the preparations: looking after myself; taking a course of reflexology; enrolling for the NCT classes, hospital birthing classes and even the local surgery's antenatal class. I read endless books on the subject, as I had had no previous experience of babies or birth or children. In fact, until I met Paul I wasn't going to have children. Up until then I had been busy with my career and hadn't given children, let alone pregnancy and birth, any great thought.

Through my research and the NCT training I realised I was a natural and active birth type! I became a fan of Sheila Kitzinger and joined up on the active birth centre web site. The NCT classes were a good focus for Paul and me to discuss all aspects of the birth and included lots of positive encouragement for active labour and birthing. We were shown lots of useful techniques with chairs, beanbags, and birthing balls. And the teacher had a great attitude to positive pain and ways of naturally controlling it. It all fed into my growing feelings about the type of birth I would like, given the choice.

One thing I found really hard to understand was why so many other pregnant women I'd met seemed to want to hand over their bodies to the medical profession and have a managed birth with as much pain relief as possible. I really believed that my body was made to do this job. I wanted that responsibility and to let it do what it was capable of doing. I wanted to let go and enjoy every minute of it and to celebrate being a woman.

Of course I could not predict how my birth would go. Maybe I would be the one in the end screaming for an epidural, but it was not what I wanted. The idea of positive pain, with a beginning, middle and a baby at the end, was something I could cope with. I spent loads of time thinking about and reading around the subject. It was instinctive to psych myself up and prepare myself mentally for pain. In hindsight this did help me get through both births with no pain relief except a little gas and air in hospital.

Not feeling confident enough to have the home birth the first time round we decided a good compromise would be to spend as much time at home during the first stages of labour as possible and just go in to hospital for the final stages and the actual birth. So we had our plan and this is what we did.

I woke up at about four o'clock on Christmas morning with mild period-like pains and thought, 'Here we go. This could be it.' There didn't seem much point in waking Paul at this stage. I wanted him as rested as possible. So I stayed in bed and waited to see how things went, but it wasn't long before I was convinced that labour had started and I decided to get up. I spent quite a while by myself getting my head around what was happening. At about 6am I wanted company and got Paul out of bed.

While Paul was packing the car and buttering sandwiches I did lots of moving and rocking curled in a ball on the floor in the early stages. I also found that, as the lower back pain increased, pressing my lower back into the handrail on the landing really helped to counter the pain.

Then as things progressed I took to our new large bath. Being submerged and buoyant relieved a lot of pressure. This was a great comfort to me now the contractions were getting progressively stronger. I realised I didn't want to be massaged or touched at this point. It was like all my senses were switched on full. Even the smell of Paul's cup of coffee was revolting.

I have always had an attraction to water and have always been a good swimmer. The water enveloped me, helped me through the pain and helped me relax fully in between the contractions. I felt that the water helped make the contractions and relaxation a unified process. It helped me focus in on myself, work with the pain during contractions and make the most of the relaxation in between. The water enabled me to leave the outside world and concentrate on the job in hand. I was in my own water world!

I cannot remember how long I was in the bath but there was no stopping this labour. It was getting faster and stronger. Paul was recording the length and strength of contractions and wondering whether we should head off into hospital. I was very reluctant to leave that bath but he realised that if we were going to make it he had to get me out. The rest is a bit of a blur.

I was nearing the last stages of labour. At that point I really hadn't come to terms with how fast it was all going. I think my overriding feelings were of irritation at having to move to get to the hospital. I was also conscious that Paul had started to panic slightly as he was probably more aware of the gravity of the situation and his responsibilities. We had heard so many stories about long labours that the speed of events threw both of us.

I was trying to stay calm but the intense focus I had had was broken. Being out of the bath felt so harsh after the confines of the water and the bathroom. It was Christmas Day morning. I was stood on our doorstep in soggy pyjamas (my waters had broken), wondering how I was ever going to get into the car and to the hospital.

Somehow we got there and were shown to the delivery suite. I vividly remember the midwife asking questions about the story so far while I was having excruciating contractions. She seemed very uninterested, almost dismissive. When she asked me to 'hop on the bed' to be monitored I nearly punched her. I don't know how I got up there or how the midwife gave me an internal but she realised I wasn't overdoing it and that I was 9cm dilated. Funnily enough her attitude changed after that.

Even fully dilated I still had to be strapped to a monitor and lie on the bed. Both these things were highly uncomfortable. My instinct by this stage was to move around and squat. I was offered gas and air, which I eagerly took, to help me through this procedure. During this monitoring Alex's heart beat started to fluctuate. The obstetrician was called and the atmosphere changed. She was concerned about the irregular heartbeat and decided Alex needed to be born as soon as possible. We managed to negotiate an hour to do this before they would intervene.

There was a panic situation going on. I was concerned about Alex's safety so for that hour I pushed for dear life. The head kept appearing during contractions and pushing but he was not coming out. In the end Alex was delivered with the help of a ventouse suction cap. The whole labour had taken eight hours.

In hindsight I think my body had stopped labour to get out of the bath and to hospital. I was fully dilated and Alex was ready to be born but my body wasn't ready. This would explain the changes in his heartbeat. I had no natural urges to push in hospital and now that I look back over the turn of events I feel sure that he would have been born very easily at home in the bath.

However, I was not disappointed with the choices we made and under the circumstances the hospital staff did everything they could. Even in the rush and panic of things the midwife was responsive to my birth plan. And when things got difficult the doctor was open to negotiating an hour of trying to push Alex out before assisting.

So even though things hadn't gone quite to plan I had still given birth to a beautiful baby boy. What a fantastic and bizarre Christmas. I have lasting memories of sunlight streaming in through the window, catching the contours of Alex's blond hair while I breastfed for the first time, Paul eating a Christmas dinner on his lap by the side of us and the Salvation Army brass band playing 'Oh little town of Bethlehem' in the corridor.

It was one of the biggest achievements of my life. I felt wonderful and so pleased with myself. What an amazing day!

Frank, 2002

There was absolutely no doubt in my mind that I wanted a home birth for my second child and if possible a water birth. I had been very pleased with how Alex's labour had gone at home and his near-delivery in the bath confirmed that water played an important part in my labour. So when I found out I was pregnant in June 2001 I made an appointment with Julie, my midwife, to discuss planning a home birth.

She was very receptive to this and had attended many women at home. She made me feel comfortable about my choice and she treated a home birth as normal as a hospital birth. I felt fully supported and we both hoped she would be the one to deliver Frank. However, when I mentioned the idea of getting a birthing pool and the possibility of giving birth under water, I was surprised to find that she had only assisted one water birth while studying twenty years earlier. This wasn't a problem, as such, but there would have to be a midwife present with water birth experience. For the first time I realised how few women use water for labour and birth. To me it was the most natural and logical thing in the world.

I was a bit nervous about seeing the doctor. I was concerned about my age. I knew that being 39 made me an old mother according to the medical profession. I wondered if I would come up against any resistance to having a home birth. Would my miscarriages and Alex's assisted birth affect her attitude towards it? I need not have been worried and, although she wasn't as supportive as I'd have liked, I think she knew I was genuinely confident and determined about having a home birth.

Our family was supportive about our plans. My mother in law, Eileen, was very interested. It brought up memories of her own births and how she would have loved to have had Paul at home but couldn't because of complications. However, they were all bemused and intrigued by the idea of the pool and giving birth in it. This wasn't an option for my mother's generation and so it must have sounded a bit strange and modern. They all wanted to know exactly how it was going to work and all showed concern about the baby coming out into water. Would he breathe in water or get water in his lungs?

I explained the procedure to them and reassured them that Frank would be fine and that his lungs would only inflate and he would start to breathe when he made contact with the air when he'd come to the surface. There was very little chance of water going into his lungs. I hope I convinced them that it would be a lovely gentle way for him to enter the world and that it would be very beneficial to me for labouring too.

I had lots of support from friends and it helped having a couple of friends who had experience of using water in labour and had hired pools from the Active Birth Centre. I found out what their births had been like, how to get hold of a pool and some useful tips. The Active Birth Centre was really helpful and ran a very organised and efficient pool hire service.

The pool arrived three weeks before my due date. We had lots of excited talks about where best to put it and which floor would be strong enough. Our friends came and joined in the construction and excitement. I really wanted it in our kitchen so I could have a lovely view of the garden – A great focus for a calm labour. As it worked out the kitchen was the best place practically too. It was close to the hot water supply and a wall underneath the floor meant it could support the weight.

Again I really enjoyed my pregnancy with Frank. I felt confident and secure in the knowledge that my body could do its thing again in an environment that was familiar and comfortable. I think Paul felt much more involved this time, practically and emotionally. We were creating our own little nesting environment together and getting giggly and excited about it. I felt very supported by him.

He was pleased that I was so confident about wanting a water birth; my confidence told him it was the right thing to do. I think he was pleased to have the job of getting the pool together and making sure it all was functioning and ready. It was something practical he could contribute towards the birth. This time I wasn't going to be just another patient in hospital giving birth. This time I knew I could deal with the labour pain without medical intervention in the privacy of my own home. I could move around, make a cup of tea, read a book (not quite!), and be free to go with my instincts. A wonderful thought! And that is pretty much what happened.

On the morning of 9 February, at around 7am, I started with gentle labour pains, and straight away Paul phoned Julie. We arranged for the grandparents to pick Alex up. He was only two at that time and we felt it might be quite frightening for him to see me in pain. Besides, I didn't want either of us distracted by having to look after him. Paul then filled the pool and Alex and I dived in for a last cuddle and chat before he became a big brother. This was a lovely time for me filled with anticipation and excitement. I didn't feel any fear or anxiety just the warmth of the water and comfort.

After we had said our goodbyes to Alex, Julie arrived. I was so pleased that she was on her shift and was able to attend my birth. It was important to me that I had some consistency: someone you know in your own home. We were lucky.

At that point she suggested I got out of the pool so she could check me. I remember Julie and I talking about how the effects of the water can speed things up. This was not what I wanted considering the speed of Alex's birth and the fact that statistically second births are faster. So I climbed out and went upstairs to move around and use the handrail again. Julie got her gear set up and made herself at home reading a book in the lounge. It was very hands off. The atmosphere was very relaxed.

It wasn't long again before the contractions became stronger and closer together. It was starting to feel like this labour was going to be at the same pace as before if not faster. I think it was then that Julie gave me an internal and said I was 4cm dilated. I was now in some pain so Paul topped up the pool and

I re-entered it. It was such a relief to feel buoyant again. I felt so relaxed that everything started to progress really fast just like Alex's labour.

Again I was able to use the water to focus in on myself, go with the pain and relax as much as possible in between contractions. Paul was always there for hand-squeezing and talking me gently through it. I remember his voice became a lovely music in the background. Julie, in the meantime, had phoned the other midwife to come ASAP. Her suspicions about a speedy birth were being confirmed.

When the second midwife arrived I was well into labour and approaching second stage. It was then that I started to feel a bit tense. It all was going too fast and I felt as if I was losing control. Julie wanted to examine me and I found it difficult to raise my body out of the water. I am not sure if she managed to check me. I think then some doubt crept into my mind as to whether I could do this.

Julie and Paul were brilliant. They soon had me relaxed and back on track. Julie massaged my shoulders and gave me a no-nonsense pep talk. This was exactly what I needed. Then I started to feel that familiar burning sensation of reaching complete dilation. I could feel Frank moving down the birth canal. He was ready to be born.

A few contractions later, with Paul supporting me from behind, our lovely boy shot out. He really did come out with some force and went floating off on his umbilical cord. Julie had to retrieve him and pass him up to me. We cried with joy and Frank, who really looked like a Frank, breast-fed for the first time. The whole thing from first contraction to birth had taken just four hours.

After some time I handed Frank to Paul and climbed out to deliver the placenta. After the checks, and a little stitch, the midwives were soon gone, leaving us alone and happy with our new baby. At 2pm we all snuggled on the sofa to catch our breath and contemplate the joy of new life.

Early in the evening our best friends came round with a bottle of champagne to celebrate Frank's safe arrival. It was a fantastic day. We even watched *Austin Powers* on TV before the three of us went to bed.

What an amazing experience to be able to give birth in the comfort and familiarity of my own home. I had felt confident that my body could do it. I was happy to be free to labour the way I wanted and to have succeeded in getting the water birth I hoped for. It felt good to have the privacy of our home, a perfect venue. There were no rigid hospital procedures or unnecessary monitoring. No bright lights, no over-cautious doctors, no crap food, no disinfectant smells. What a great way to come into the world!

Laura's story

Lillian, 2004

When I had my first booking-in appointment and the midwife asked what hospital I'd like to go to, I said I'd like a home birth. This wasn't really based on anything tangible like experience or research, but it sounded like a nice idea. The midwife seemed surprised and went on to describe how pain relief options were limited and how it was more common for women who already had children to have home births, as they knew what to expect.

I asked the midwife about her own childbirth experiences; she said that she'd had her three babies in the hospital because she needed all pain relief options due to her low pain threshold. Oh dear, that sounded like me. She wrote up my notes and put 'home birth?' I don't think either of us at that stage thought there was much chance of it happening. I can't even remember talking to Ant, my partner, about it that much at that stage.

At 24 weeks pregnant I started NCT classes. I remember that I went alone to the first class as Ant was working, but as expected everyone was thoroughly pleasant. My only disquieting moment came when at the end of the class the discussion descended into a free-for-all against Horrid Doctors. Feeling like I might well end up in hospital with every intervention going, I challenged this view, defending the doctors and their interventionist ways. Thankfully someone backed me and I didn't feel a complete arse.

Interestingly, one of the group, whose baby was due first, was also a trainee midwife. Not only this but she was planning to have a home birth. Typical, is what I thought.

Over the next few sessions my desire for knowledge about giving birth grew nearly as big as my belly. I was happy to go to the NCT classes, sign up for hospital classes, read books, look on the internet and soak it all up. Fairly quickly I bought into the idea that birth could and should be a natural process and one to look forward to, not to dread. I began to focus on the idea of a home birth. My main concern was, what if I couldn't cope?

This was a concern that my partner shared. In the early days he was very worried about the impact it would have on me and the baby… you know, what if it goes wrong? But my confidence grew and I became clearer that I wanted a home birth. The discussions continued at home without any clear resolution and it was during this period that I started to talk more openly with friends and family about the home birth option.

I can honestly say that, with the exception of my sister, who'd had a baby the year before, the response was largely negative. Those who weren't openly negative about the idea said things like, "You wait, when you're in the throes of labour you'll need every pain relief option going," or simply asked, "What if it all goes wrong?" And everyone had a bad story to tell about giving birth; why do people do that? I felt patronised by the 'you wait and see' attitude and like a reckless risk-taker with the 'what if it goes wrong' brigade. Anthony was going to need some serious persuasion before he could really buy into the home birth option.

During one of the last NCT classes we watched a video of women giving birth. A mixture of home, water and hospital births were shown to us, none of which looked particularly appealing at 33 weeks pregnant. But the idea of labouring at home, being able to do exactly what I needed to do to get me through, became essential to me.

After the video we discussed how we felt about the births we'd watched. It was then that I raised my dilemma with the class. It was Aby (the aforementioned trainee midwife) who pointed out that if I opted for a home birth and the labour was going well I could stay at home but that at any point I could change my mind and go into hospital. If, on the other hand, I was booked for a hospital birth and the labour was going well at home I couldn't at the eleventh hour opt to stay put.

This was a revelation! Knowing that I could change my mind at any point gave us both the confidence we'd so far lacked to commit to a home birth. I should add that the fact that we live only half an hour from the hospital also helped: I'm not sure we'd have felt the same if we'd been an hour away.

Aby also pointed out that at home you get one-to-one care (in fact, when the moment arrives, there should be two midwives). This was great. I'd heard friends complain that they were often left alone to deal with contractions and my poor old sister said that she'd pushed for hours exhausting herself for lack of guidance on the matter. The fact that I'd get one-to-one attention made me feel all the more special.

As the due date got closer I started to notice a little voice in my head: it said 'You can do it, your body was made for this, women have been doing it successfully like this for centuries.' It became a little mantra and it worked. I believed it more and my confidence grew. Yes, I was anxious – birth was an unknown quantity – but I knew that this baby had to come out whatever and being positive about it made me feel stronger.

I resolved to confirm my intentions with the midwife at my next appointment. I thought I'd have a battle on my hands and I was sure she'd try and talk me out of it. Unusually my mum was there for this appointment and while she hadn't voiced a view on home births either way it seemed to somehow make a difference with the midwife. Of course I'll never know, but I just felt like she wasn't going to question my judgement with my mum there!

A week before my due date my waters broke, just after lunch. My best friend Lorna happened to be staying with us for the night having come visiting from Rome. We called the midwife even though I wasn't having contractions, to give them some advance warning, and I was introduced to the on-call midwife, Nicky, around 4pm. She came back a few hours later to assess progress. There wasn't any. She gave me some good advice and said she'd come back tomorrow unless I needed her before then.

Ant and Lorna popped out for a takeaway at about nine o'clock, by ten the contractions had started and by eleven they were steady. The TENS machine I'd hired was great for the half hour before it broke and I ditched it. By midnight the contractions were coming thick and fast. The videos of births we'd seen at NCT showed women wondering around having a cup of tea in between contractions but this was not my experience. I wanted to call Nicky but Anthony seemed a bit hesitant, so we agreed to start timing the contractions. When we realised how close they were we called her straight away: they were coming 90 seconds apart.

Nicky arrived at 12:40am and confirmed I was 4cm dilated. Pain relief came in the form of a hot water bottle and my birthing ball. I got very hot and cold quickly and Anthony was fantastic at responding to all my requests. Together, in our bedroom, we focused on the contractions and rode them out.

At around one o'clock the pain got really bad and I was still only 5cm dilated. (Five? Surely she meant twenty-five?) All I could think was if I've got another ten hours of this I can't cope and I'll have to go to the hospital. I remember having coded conversations with Nicky to this effect. To their credit Nicky and Ant kept me going.

Nicky suggested I went downstairs to have a bath. Before I got in I remember hanging onto the washbasin and retching and shuddering like a volt had gone through my body. Ant washed my back with the shower and I instantly hated it and wanted to get out. They persuaded me to give it a minute. I did and suddenly it felt wonderful, the pain eased. Nicky was great as she followed our lead and largely left us to it. I think something happened when I came down those stairs because within an hour of being in the bath I was ready to push.

I remember asking for gas and air but Nicky said that in the time it would take to set it up the baby would be here. It was then I thought: 'Okay, you've done it, home birth, no drugs, enjoy the next few minutes.'

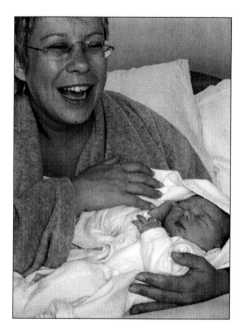

The pushing bit was so much better for me than the contractions. I felt more in control and I was getting somewhere. I could feel our baby travelling down me with every push. I remember the hot pain when she was crowning, I remember panting for my life when I had to stop pushing to allow her head to come out of its own accord. But mostly I remember being so incredibly proud of myself for having a natural home birth and giving Ant the beautiful baby we'd wanted for so long.

Lillian Rose was born at 3:25am and half an hour later we were all in our own bed having a cup of tea. An hour after that it was just the three of us (and Lorna, who had slept through most of the action). It was weeks later when Nicky told us that Lillian was her first home birth. Wow – what a great memory for all of us!

I feel incredibly lucky and privileged that the labour and birth was so textbook. And that's the issue: you just don't know what it'll be like. But for us, being so close to the hospital and having that one-to-one care during labour made it feel safe for us to take the plunge.

Did the home birth make a difference to us? For the first three months we just kept reliving it. We still do, but not quite so often. It is our most treasured memory, so far.

Karen's story

Dan, 2004

After his sister Katie's birth, Dan's was a most cathartic experience. Katie was my first child and a footling breech. She turned head-up at 38 weeks, leaving me suddenly unable to bend. No amount of acupuncture, sitting and sleeping in funny positions and external cephalic versions would shift her.

Terrified of hospitals and distrusting the medical profession, I tried to escape the horror of a planned caesarean section by leaving her as long as possible and hoping against hope that she would turn herself. She didn't. And at 42½ weeks, I signed the consent form and had her cut out. We were all fine, the operation wasn't as horrible as I expected, and recovery was frustrating but okay. But the mental scars are deep: I am still aghast at the butchery of the process and wary, knowing the additional risks to all future children.

Jon and I carried on with our plan to have our two children close together, and I was soon pregnant again, a 16-month gap between birth dates. This time, if the child was in a sensible position for the birth, wild horses wouldn't drag me to hospital – I was staying at home. I felt safer with the idea of running off to Cader Idris and giving birth with the sheep than going back to the 'butchers'. I was terrified of being dragged to hospital, having my labour freeze and undergoing a second section with a 16-month-old at home to pick up and look after.

I was now made to feel like a walking uterine scar. My community midwife said that they would support my wishes, but the undercurrent was always 'You couldn't do it last time: what makes you think you'll be able to this time?'

At ten days before due date the phone rang. "We are unlikely to be able to supply a community midwife with any home birth experience and it is February: if it is icy it will be dangerous to send one out to you…." No home birth experience?

And what about VBAC (vaginal birth after caesarean)? The supervisor of midwives had told us that they would have an ambulance waiting outside the house all the way through my labour "just in case". Of uterine rupture, that is, which can also happen to an unscarred uterus, and with a risk similar to the 'You really should have this' amniocentisis test. Nice atmosphere to give birth in. Not. So I contacted an independent midwife, Lis.

Lis arrived like a guardian angel, calm and confident. She booked me in with a week to go, suggesting a birthpool which I got locally and which we assembled in the dining room. I picked up my TENS machine and my pethidine. I was ready for anything.

On the evening before the due date I felt 'funny' every 20 minutes. Not having been in labour with Katie, I wasn't sure what was happening, so I put my TENS machine on low and went to bed. At 5am it was 'funny' every five minutes. I rolled over to go back to sleep. Jon made me get up and telephone Lis who, to my surprise, insisted on coming over immediately.

While I waited for Lis to arrive, I tidied the kitchen, emptied last night's veg peelings on the compost heap and had breakfast. At 7am Lis arrived from Lutterworth. The 'funny feeling' time interval was three minutes but no pain. She watched me for half an hour, then asked if she could have a look. "It's not labour yet, but dilation is starting." The next contraction went 'whoosh bang' – waters broken, strong contractions and away we went.

Plans were to mobilise. So much for plans. I knelt on the floor, leant over the seat of the sofa and fell asleep. Three minutes later... Oh! There's another one, just like the other one! Contraction over, I fell asleep. By 9:30am I was desperate for Jon to take Katie to nursery and climb into the birthing pool, but that meant taking off my beloved TENS machine – dilemma!

I climbed into the pool saying, "That last one was unpleasant," and Lis said, "Push on the next one." Push? I couldn't be there yet could I? I leant against the side of the pool and dozed, waiting. The pattern was set: cramp in my belly, big breath in, reach for the gas and air, big breath out through the mouthpiece, a satisfying walrus sound, "Sorry, I forgot to push. I'll do it next time," doze over the side of the pool.

At some point a second midwife, Sarah, appeared from out of the ether (aka Birmingham). I slept through my two-hour hospital limit for the 2nd stage, but heart rates for me and mine were steady and strong, I was still fresh (no wonder after all that sleep) and the contractions were still strong.

The worst bit was when the head descended. I suddenly wanted to lean back, but was too short to reach the other side of the pool. I struggled to keep my head above water. "Jon, stop me from drowning. Get in the pool." He dared to pause to take off his trousers: what audacity! There wasn't time for such niceties! Lis, however, was impressed that he'd actually climbed into the pool with me.

Dan was born at 1:10pm. All 8lb 14oz of him. I had a bruised cheek from all that dozing. Twenty minutes later, I was eating Battenburg cake and drinking tea on the sofa with my parents arriving to tell me, "You can't have fish and chips; you've just had a baby!" Well, I still had a placenta to deliver too, but that could wait until it was eventually persuaded to depart with a homeopathic treatment of some sort.

Katie came home about an hour later, able to sit on her mummy's lap without being pushed off by a hard tummy. She was chuffed about that, but completely nonplussed about her baby brother, whom she now adores. All we need now is the dog I'd been promised for having our own babies... and of course to say thanks to everyone who gave me encouragement – thank you.

For another perspective on this experience, you can read Jon's story on p.249

Lucy's story

Oscar, 2005

I first thought about having a home birth when I was pregnant with my daughter, but my midwife was discouraging and so my husband, Bod, was anxious about the idea too. I ended up with a hospital delivery with an epidural and forceps which was exactly what I hadn't wanted; I had not received good advice or support from the hospital team.

When pregnant with my son I didn't give the idea much thought until my sister asked if I would be having a home birth and a close friend, Sarah, suggested it too. When I first spoke to my midwife, Joanne, about it she seemed aloof and said there wasn't much point going into details early on as so many factors could prevent make a home birth. So I crossed my fingers and hoped.

Bod was again a little anxious about the idea, not least because we had new carpets downstairs! My friend Sarah was training to be an antenatal teacher and so was very up-to-date on every aspect of labour and birth. She was a wonderful source of information, encouragement and help. Plus I was under no illusion that if it went like my daughter's birth had (slowly) I would be straight off to hospital for drugs. But I felt strongly that I must try to do it 'properly'.

I also felt that when I'd had my daughter in hospital the staff were so busy dealing with other women that I was mistaken for someone else and not given more options to manage my pain. I felt if I stayed at home with just one midwife, she couldn't confuse me with anyone else, would know everything that had happened to me, and would be better equipped to give me appropriate advice.

Most people's reaction to me telling them I was planning a home birth was, "Aren't you brave?" This response baffled me as I was not doing it for reasons of bravery, more for selfish reasons. Mine and Bod's families didn't really comment except for my sister who was jealous as she had been induced for both of her children and loved the idea of a home birth.

Friends were supportive and interested in my reason. So much so that one friend decided to go for it, and had a wonderful home birth herself as I'd given such a good argument! Some people thought I was mad, but mostly I was met with support. I did enjoy, when people asked where I would be having my baby, saying "At home" and checking their reactions.

My pregnancy was very healthy and as the weeks flew by I began to talk to my midwife in more detail about the home birth. She still didn't commit to discussing it in full until she dropped off the kit at my house when I was 35 weeks, by which time she was very supportive. I was able to see her point of view with the possibility of things changing but felt a little disappointed about her dismissing it week after week.

A student midwife on placement with my midwife lived locally to me and asked if she could attend the birth, and I was happy for her to do so. I had also suggested half jokingly to my friend Sarah that she ought to attend a birth to be able to teach about them, although when she offered seriously to be present I was a little unsure. But as the weeks went on I was glad of the support because Sarah really knew what she was talking about when it came to giving birth (plus she'd had two children herself).

We had made provisions for Alice to be looked after in a number of ways in all the different situations. One was that a friend would take time off work to look after Alice; another that my dad would travel over from Shropshire; a third that Sarah would look after her with her boys. My ideal was for the whole thing to happen at night and for Alice to sleep through it: wishful thinking I guess.

Things began to get a little worrying when my due date came and went. The hospital had moved my due date forward by ten days at the twelve-week scan and, on reaching a week overdue, my midwife tried to book me in for an induction. This, along with a c-section, was my worst fear and I told her I would refuse to be induced unless they could give me a better reason than just that their dates said so.

My midwife, Joanne, said that I would have to visit the consultant to which I agreed. I said I would be induced, but only a week after my own due date not theirs (according to my own cycle I wasn't due for another three days). Joanne booked me in to see the consultant but also did a cervical sweep at home. She told me on first exam that my cervix was totally shut and it would be very difficult to do a 'good sweep' but she would try. I told her to go for it, and she agreed but told me it would probably be quite uncomfortable. It was very painful but if it worked it would be worth it.

Joanne said she had a good feeling about it as she had done a good one so Amanda (her student) and I crossed our fingers. I was told to expect abdominal pains and discomfort as a result of the sweep, and to go out for a hilly walk to help get things moving about. I spent the afternoon at Sarah's house feeling very down about the idea of induction and quite uncomfortable.

When my husband came home I was really feeling low and fed up, but went out with some friends and their dog to a local country park for a very hilly walk. At one point I was so tired I went onto all fours so I could breathe. My friends were a little concerned but I insisted we kept going – I was determined to shift this baby! While we were out Bod had cooked dinner and put Alice, who was nearly three, to bed.

We finished our lovely meal and sat down for the evening and I felt really very uncomfortable and wondered if it was the start of labour. We knew we would soon find out. I had a hot bath and listened to a relaxation CD Sarah had given me specifically for labour and birth and as I lay in the bath visualising contractions I began to realise I was actually experiencing them for real. When I got out of the bath we put on the TENS machine and I thought I had better go to bed and try to rest as much as possible.

I did get Bod to look at the clock when I got uncomfortable, and we realised the pains definitely came and went, and were about seven minutes apart. I didn't really sleep but did rest a bit. It was 11pm before it got too much for me to lay still and so I went downstairs and rang the duty midwife as instructed. I was told by the midwife that she was from the team that covered our area every other day so she would have to travel twenty minutes to get to assess me. I wasn't in any panic, but as it was my second child she felt she had better come and see me. Amanda was called and I rang Sarah to let her know. She came immediately over followed shortly by Amanda.

I left Bod in bed, thinking there was little need to wake him as there was no point in him being up when nothing was really going on. Plus, if Alice did need looking after, I didn't want him to be tired and short tempered. The contractions were strong but not really painful and I was managing to chat with Sarah and Amanda in between and going onto all fours for each contraction. I felt ill and vomited, then the midwife arrived and Sarah was wonderful and made drinks for everyone.

I used a variety of positions, helped by Sarah. I had a big gym ball which I had used to sit on in pregnancy, but found putting my arms over it and rocking most comfortable. We discussed that I wasn't resting enough in between contractions when on the floor with the ball. I found the decision difficult to make, as using the ball was excellent during the contractions, but when my contractions became stronger I lay down on the sofa and buried my face in Sarah's fleece top.

The midwife was holding my stomach and feeling the contractions to assess where I was. I had some very strong, quite painful ones and some funny sort of half ones, but she was happy that my progress was good and decided that they had better stay with me if it carried on going so well.

I was getting restless on the sofa and, not wanting to go upstairs and wake Alice, we pulled out the guest sofa bed in the living room and I climbed on there. I carried on hugging Sarah tightly round her middle. Feeling very calm and in control I did a lot of deep breathing and letting go with the outward breath which I found incredibly helpful.

Things seemed to be going well, but the contractions were getting stronger and I had been missing Bod, so at 1am I asked Sarah to get him up. Funnily enough he had heard my louder contractions and was getting up anyway! Sarah had got everything I had needed and Bod was stunned to see how far along I had gone; he hadn't realised how long he had been asleep.

The midwife said she would have to do an internal exam to see how I was getting on. She had not done one up to then, but as the practice was to get a second midwife in for the delivery, plus with the neighbouring team being on call, she wanted to leave time to be organised. Bod lay down on the bed with me and I was so pleased to have him there. With him behind me and Sarah in front I felt so secure physically and mentally. I was ready for anything!

Before starting the exam Sarah suggested I have some gas and air, which I was grateful for, and when the midwife did the exam and told me I was at least 7 or 8 cm dilated we were all shocked (and

I was delighted!). Then my waters broke, and my final anxiety of having to be transferred to hospital was gone as the midwife told me the waters were fine. I remember asking, "Is there meconium? Is there meconium?" I was also shocked at how much water there was... and hoping it didn't go on the carpet!

Then I was overwhelmed with fear and panic as it dawned on me that this was real and I was going to have to have this baby, here in my living room, with no epidural and lots of pain! I lay on the bed saying to Sarah and Bod, "I can't do this," and I really meant it. Sarah smiled a big wide smile and I knew she was thinking I was in transition. I remember thinking so clearly, 'But I am *not* in transition – I *can't do this*!'

Then, after everyone telling me I could do it, the midwife told me I might need to push soon. She hadn't been able to get another midwife in to help so Amanda, the student, was called on to assist her. Thankfully I had plenty of help. So, again on Sarah's suggestion, I was recommended to be more upright. The gym ball was lifted up onto the bed where I put my arms over it and knelt up, then I had the overwhelming urge to push, and pushed for all my life was worth with Bod holding my hands and encouraging me.

I remember everyone shouting at me: it seemed very distant and it took what felt like a while to hear. I was confused because I thought you had to pant when delivering the baby's head, and I was waiting for the burning, awful pain people talk about, but next push I felt the most incredible pressure release and I knew it was over.

I was so relieved and so pleased I had done it, that when I heard Sarah's voice telling me it was a boy I felt like: 'Who cares what sex it is?' I was so tired, and so pleased. I turned to hold him and saw this beautiful little face and felt so much love for my son. Bod and I were really shocked as we were both convinced I was having another girl.

We decided immediately on the name Oscar. He was born at 3:45am weighing 9lb 11oz. Oscar had got his shoulders stuck on the way out, and the midwife was concerned with the size of the tear I had, and wanted me to go to hospital for stitches. At this suggestion I got very upset, so we were given a bit more time to digest this. We rang our relatives and looked at our new boy: he was perfect.

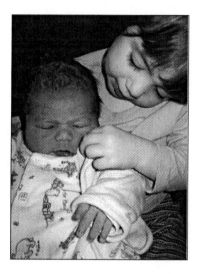

The midwife decided that the tear did need to be seen to in hospital so arranged for an ambulance to take me in. Sarah came with me so that Bod could stay with Alice. He woke her up at 5am so she could see her new baby before we went to hospital; she was tired but very excited to see her new baby had arrived. I got myself together and went to the hospital. The stitches were worse than the delivery, but I was so glad to only have to go in for stitches not during labour.

Bod helped clear up the mess (he threw away the mattress from the sofa bed!) and I was home again in two hours, by which time my dad had come over to help with Alice for the day.

Having had the home birth was amazing. Alice slept through everything just as I had hoped. It had been quick and I had felt in control and empowered by it. I had been very lucky to get incredible support from Sarah and Bod and to have such an experienced midwife. It was so good to have such consistent care during the birth and it was magical to be at home right away and for Alice to spend such wonderful time with her new brother. I felt so much more comfortable being at home with my new baby afterwards: in my own bed, on my own sofa and with my own family.

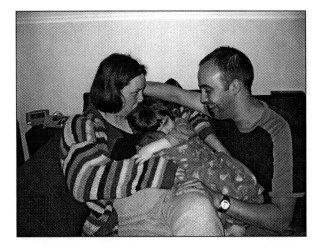

I think the experience brought us closer as a family. I feel that there have been so many positives, the only negative thing I could think of was that I didn't have the name tickets from baby's hand and foot from hospital for a memory box. Everything else has been simply amazing, and there is nothing more I could have hoped for. It was honestly the perfect birth.

Kris's stories

James, 1997

As soon as I found out I was pregnant I knew I wanted a home birth. For me there just didn't seem to be a better place. Hospitals are for sick people aren't they?

I researched the subject in preparation for meeting the midwife. I was expecting fierce opposition as that seemed to be the pattern of the vast majority of accounts I'd read. But, much to my delight, a very supportive community midwife agreed that home births are not the norm in this country but are completely safe. We agreed I would double book so that if there was any reason for a transfer to hospital during labour or delivery we wouldn't have to waste time filling in paperwork.

Things were going well until my routine hospital appointment. I had my first scan and everything was fine. But because we'd declined the screening tests I was given an appointment with a registrar. We were subjected to a twenty-minute session of bullying by him and the clinic nurse. "What happens if the baby is born with a defect?" "What if you bleed heavily?" "Why should an ambulance attend because you *chose* not to be in hospital?" This was the last thing we needed.

In the end, I refused to come back for my second scan and was crying so much the clinic receptionist arranged to get the consultant to see us. He was surprisingly supportive. His attitude was that he'd worked in the inner city USA where he'd seen babies born in the most unsuitable conditions with no complications: so with a clean house and proper care by trained midwives we were not at a very increased risk.

As we were leaving we noticed the same registrar looking very sheepish as we passed him and the consultant in the corridor having a very intense discussion. Perhaps he was converted? Or at least learned to respect personal choice that day.

So… on with the birth. I wasn't due for another two weeks so we decided to go to a friend's birthday party. The other half had rather a lot to drink that evening. But it's a first baby, not due for fifteen days, first babies are notoriously late, etc, etc. He really pushed the boat out.

We returned at 3am the following morning following a very speedy taxi journey over very large speed bumps. I felt a bit sore when we got in and decided to go straight to bed. I got up two hours later to go to the loo, as was the nightly custom, and was about to get back into bed when I felt a trickle down my leg. I immediately attempted to wake my other half without a great deal of success, so decided as no one else was too concerned, and I wasn't in any pain, I'd go back to bed.

I wasn't able to sleep much and finally got up with a back-ache at six o'clock. I rang the midwife at nine and she popped round. Nothing much doing, so she went away again and I got on with my day. We went into town to fetch the pram, went to the shops and I carried on as normal as possible with niggling contractions and wearing extra-large disposable nappies in my knickers to catch my waters as they coped better than mater-nity towels. The midwife came back in the afternoon and I was still only 2-3cm dilated so we had the in-laws round to tea as planned and went out for another walk.

Things were getting more painful by now, so I went to have a shower and was in there for an hour or so. At 10pm, the midwife rang. Did we need her? No, not yet, as things were still bearable. We settled down for a long night watching *Men Behaving Badly* on video. Contractions slowed from every five minutes to every seven or eight minutes around midnight, which was a relief as I'd been having backache the entire time. At 3am we went for a walk as things were starting to pick up again. At 5am I rang the midwife. Still 3cm. The midwife worked out that he was lying back to back so he had to turn around as well, which was why it was so slow and the backache was there.

At 7am the midwife came out again to give the number of her replacement as she was off duty now. We went walking again as it was a gloriously warm and sunny day at the beginning of March. My mother-in-law and sister-in-law came round later to visit and by midday I was feeling very tired. We rang the new midwife and she came over and stayed with us.

She was just as fantastic as the last one, encouraging me to change position and use gravity to bring his head round, making drinks and supporting my by now very tired and shell-shocked other half. The contractions were now every three to four minutes and were double-peaking, which was very hard to deal with.

The next four hours are a blur, but then a new midwife came and checked my urine as I was exhausted. I was in ketosis so she made me tea with three sugars and toast with so much honey on I can't bear to eat it to this day nearly nine years later! But it worked and my energy levels picked up a bit. She was rather bossy and ran a bath that I really didn't want to get into. She marched me upstairs, which I didn't want to do, and put me in the bath – and what blessed relief! The pain was nowhere near as intense as it had been. Thank God for bossy midwives!

By 6pm the gas and air came out as I had finally progressed to 6cm. What great pain relief I found it. I was falling asleep in the bath between contractions which by now were every three minutes. By 7pm I'd used nearly all the gas and air so an ambulance crew came out and brought a fresh one. I can vividly remember them waiting on the stairs for me to finish the old one so they could take it back with them. At 7:30pm the second midwife was called, and arrived quickly.

Around 8pm I started pushing. I was still in the bath at this point and the midwives were happy to leave me in there. Unfortunately I stood up to move round and slipped, so I had to get out, which I wanted to do even less than I'd wanted to get in in the first place. The midwives helped me out and put a dust sheet and towels on the bed and I waddled in and heaved my great bulk onto the bed.

Within fifteen minutes of pushing as my body told me to, my 6lb 13oz baby was delivered with a second degree tear. I chose to have a natural third stage, the placenta was delivered ten minutes later and I was stitched up. That was the most painful bit of the whole birth for me. The midwives cleared up and were on their way by 10pm. My in-laws came round to meet their first grandchild and we opened the champagne. I managed one sip and fell off to sleep while everyone else celebrated around me.

A few days later a midwife was reading my notes and commented on how lucky I was to have chosen a home delivery. She reckoned had I been in hospital I would have had my labour artificially accelerated; as my son was posterior he might have gotten stuck and would have been a caesarean section because my waters had been broken over 24 hours. But at home the midwives did minimal internals and just took my temperature every two hours to keep an eye on it in case of infection from my waters breaking early. After hearing these words I felt so pleased that I'd followed my instinct and birthed at home.

Kieran, 1999

My next birth couldn't have been more different. I was twelve days overdue and the midwife rang in the morning to see if anything was happening: I hadn't even had the slightest twinge. In fact, only the day before his head had still been free. I was under threat of hospital induction in a day's time so I was feeling pretty desperate.

I had been told castor oil could help things along so I duly took half the bottle. Nothing. Then I remembered that golden-seal tincture is said to help tip the balance if things are ready, so at 6pm I took a teaspoonful and repeated that every half hour until 8pm. Nothing. I put son number one to bed and decided to go myself not long after.

At 8:15pm the castor oil kicked in and my insides felt all wrong. At 8:30 I felt the first definite contraction after taking a final dose of castor oil and goldenseal. The next few hours are a haze of going to the loo rather a lot and having contractions. I wasn't sure which were which but figured I had hours to go yet after last time.

At 12:15am we rang the midwife answering service and they got the midwife to ring us back. After speaking to me she decided to venture out and said she'd be twenty minutes or so. By 12:25 the contractions were getting unbearable and there was no midwife in sight. I was on all fours in the kitchen with my head on the floor trying to relieve the urge to push. My waters hadn't broken yet so I could just about cope.

At 12:40am the midwife arrived and as she was bringing her things in from the car my waters broke. Meanwhile I was saying some rather unladylike things about how quickly the gas and air had better appear and the poor midwife was trying to explain that she hadn't had time to set it up. As soon as she brought the last thing in from the car and knelt down beside me, the baby's head appeared and two minutes later his body, all 8lb 15 ½ oz, shot out. She turned to my other half and laughed that if there'd been any traffic he'd have been delivering the baby and not her.

Again I had a natural third stage and almost immediately the placenta appeared. Then I was stitched up, as I'd torn in the same place as last time. This time I was quite anaemic (I had been just slightly first time round), so they kept a closer eye on my blood loss at delivery. But it was minimal and we were able to stay at home as planned. My older son slept through everything and woke up the next morning to find he had a brother.

We didn't ring my in-laws straight away this time as it was late, but the next day when we rang my mother-in-law asked if he'd been born at 12:47. When we said he had, she told us that she hadn't been able to sleep and that was the last time she looked at the clock before she fell asleep. We hadn't rung to let them know I was in labour that night either. I guess it's just women's intuition or some primal connection but it's certainly very strange.

Merrin, 2002

Merrin was a day early. I was due on 30 January and with having had one early and the next late I wasn't sure when she'd be born, but I wasn't holding my breath.

The pregnancy was definitely not as easy as the other two: I had all-day sickness for thirty weeks. This left me quite anaemic but not really symptomatic with it. I found that iron in tablet or liquid form makes me very ill, so I was prescribed Spatone iron which I took for the last eight weeks three times a day. It seemed to help a little.

My midwife and I had a very good relationship by now as she'd delivered my oldest and looked after me through the other two pregnancies, so we agreed that she'd get advice from the consultant at the hospital where I was double booked. The consultant advised her to get blood sent off to be typed and cross-matched in case of a bleed at delivery, but he was still in agreement with me trying for a home delivery as long as I was aware of the risks.

I woke on the morning of the 29th feeling tired. I took my oldest to school and dropped Kieran off at playgroup, then went home and was slightly sick, which wasn't unusual as I'd spent my entire pregnancy with my head down the loo. I decided to sleep for an hour and woke up feeling better.

Kieran came home and had some lunch. I wasn't feeling much like eating and felt slightly odd; I decided I must be coming down with something. Kieran went to play with my mother-in-law as I had a midwife appointment that day. I went to the midwife having what I thought were the same Braxton-Hicks contractions I'd been having for months, but these were comparatively mild so I thought nothing of it. When I got there I told her about the niggles and that I had to keep going to the loo as I was sure I needed a wee, but when I got there I didn't. She decided these were contractions and that, with hindsight, the ones I'd been having for months probably were as well.

I was 5cm dilated when she examined me and the only way she would let me go home was if I called my other half to come back. I agreed and went to my mother-in-law's to ask her to pick up my older son. I tidied up and carried on as normal when my friend came with her children for tea as it was already arranged and I didn't feel that I needed to cancel. My other half was at home by then. I learned later that I'd scuppered his trip to the pub and presentation of baby things when I rang him at work.

Had I been any later I wouldn't have been able to reach him and he might have missed it all.

My friend made tea for the children while he and I went for a walk – it was getting hard to concentrate with everyone in the house. At 5:30pm we rang the on-call midwife. She had to come up the M1 at rush hour so she was going to be a while. She asked us to ring the ambulance if things picked up before she got there.

My friend and her children left at six and my boys were taken away for the night a bit later. I got in the bath and the midwife arrived at 6:25pm. I was coping well and when she examined me my waters broke (all over the duvet unfortunately). At seven o'clock I was 8cm and still coherent. My other half made himself and the midwife a coffee and they came into the room to drink it. I must have been in transition by then because the smell was so overpowering I asked them to drink it in the hall.

At 7:27 I got up to go for a wee, got halfway across my room and shouted for the midwife to get the plastic down. My 8lb 4oz daughter was born two minutes later; I had to support her as the midwife got her gloves on, she came out that quickly. Again, I had a natural third stage and the placenta was delivered in five minutes or so with minimal bleeding.

The midwife helped me get in the bath and then set about taking things to the car, sorting the bed out and finding fresh blankets and sleeping bags for us. When she came back in I'd gotten myself out of the bath, got dressed and was phoning people to let them know the baby was here. Her grandparents met her when she was only three hours old, and the only reason it was that long was because my father-in-law had been out playing badminton and was uncontactable. My boys were so excited when they came back in the morning and Merrin went with us to take them to school. I felt so well.

Gabriel, 2004

Gabriel's birth has a bit of a comedy factor but I'm sure it'll be years before he sees the funny side of it.

Again I was very anaemic so we just assumed that that's how my body will get each pregnancy: it quickly rights itself afterwards. Gabriel was born on his due date. The midwife came round at 10:30 in the morning and there was nothing happening so she gave me an appointment for the following week.

The kids were still on school holidays so everyone was at home. I took my daughter to get her hair cut in the morning while my other half stayed with the boys. He went to work in the afternoon because nothing was going on. The boys watched a video and Merrin fell asleep and so did I.

At 4pm the boys went to martial arts class with their grandma and shortly after that I had my first contraction. I put Merrin in the bath to play so I could keep an eye on her but not have to do too much. The boys came home around 8pm and my other half was very late from work. I wasn't able to contact him so their dad stayed until he got home. I watched *Raiders of the Lost Ark* on telly as a way of distracting myself between contractions on all fours on the living room floor.

The boys went to bed but Merrin wouldn't. At 8:15 my other half got home – he'd been stuck in town waiting for buses. By this time I was sure I was in labour but not needing the midwife yet. At 9:45 I ran a bath and got in, but my daughter was still up and making it difficult to concentrate. I couldn't decide if I wanted the midwife yet. I got a bit tearful and decided it was probably a good idea as I was in the bath and didn't want to get out by then or speak to anyone.

We rang my mother-in-law who picked Merrin up to go to her house for the night. I think she sensed something was happening and wouldn't go to bed. The midwife only lived ten minutes away, so she was at our house by 10:30pm. I was 8cm dilated by then but still feeling okay. I just pottered about between contractions until 10.50, then I needed a wee so I got up and went to the loo. I sat down and couldn't work out why I couldn't go.

The midwife was just outside the door, which was lucky, because all of a sudden I felt a churning sensation and shouted to her. My waters broke then and my other half got me to stand up; Gabriel was born at 10.55pm over the loo and the placenta followed swiftly after. Absolutely no mess to clean up as it all went down the loo! I had a shower and then went to bed. The boys woke up the next morning to their first day back at school and a new brother who went on his first school run at ten hours old.

I don't think we can underestimate the power of choice and responsibility for our own bodies and birth. Or the part this plays in the subsequent bonding with our new babies and their siblings with them. If they are happy to be there (awake or asleep) and mum is happy to have them there, I think it's beneficial for siblings to see the new baby as an immediate member of the family and not someone responsible for taking mummy away. And birth does not mean them going to stay somewhere else when they must already feel confused and insecure.

I hope this book will help to change the attitudes of the vast majority, who are too scared or view home birth as irresponsible, to see that we are a very aware group of people who make the decision to birth where we feel safest and happiest. I was so surprised by the opposition I encountered the first two times from family, friends and complete strangers. And at times I found it quite a lonely decision, even though I knew with all my heart it was the right one for my family. If my four very different births offer comfort or affirmation to just one woman, who then goes on to deliver at home and passes that joy on by telling her story to others, then I will feel I've made a real difference.

Since sharing my birth stories with friends one has gone on to have a successful home birth after two unpleasant hospital experiences and another tried but transferred in after complications developed. Both say they never would have contemplated home delivery if they hadn't known someone who had done it first and was willing to share their experiences. I am so excited to be sharing my stories in this book and hope it gives people the confidence to birth in the most natural environment.

For another perspective on this experience, you can read Robin's story on p.255

Sarah O's story

Lauren, 2004

I was all prepared to have my first baby in hospital, mainly because my doctor steered me that way. As I hate hospitals, and we don't have a local one, I asked my midwife how soon after giving birth I could be discharged. She said, "All being well, six hours. Why?" When I explained, she suggested a home birth: I'd had no problems during my pregnancy and it should be fine as long as my blood pressure didn't go up.

My husband was so pleased as he didn't have to worry about getting me to hospital on time and having to travel to visit. And I felt a lot more relaxed about the whole idea of childbirth now: it was like having a weight lifted off my shoulders. When I mentioned my choice to the doctor he wasn't too keen as it was my first pregnancy and only three weeks to my due date, but there was no changing my mind. It helped that my midwife, Doreen, was so helpful, supportive and informative from beginning to end.

As my due date came and went, I can't describe how fed up and uncomfortable I was. I would have tried anything to get the baby out. Ten days over and to top it off my midwife was away: her relief sent me to the hospital in Warwick to be induced. I was gutted.

We arrived at 8:30am on 23 March. I was shown to a bed, strapped to a monitor then left for half an hour. I had no internal examination as they were busy on labour ward. The nurse came back and said there were three ladies in front of me so I would have to wait. I felt like I was on a production line.

Four hours passed and still no news. Then finally I was told it would probably be the next morning before they could induce me. Well, that was no good for me, so we asked if I could go home and come back: I think they were so relieved they said okay and asked me to come back in two days time.

At 8:30 the next day we got up and I had a very unusual pain I couldn't describe. I told Wayne I thought I had a contraction and the response was, "Oh well, wait to see if you have another to be sure." He put a shower curtain on the sofa and carried on watching the telly. *Great!*

So I sat and timed the contractions. According to all the books they come in gradually and take some time before you should contact the midwife. Well, it didn't work out like that for me. I was waiting until they were five minutes apart as guided by the books, and was rather shocked when they went straight down from eighteen minutes to one minute apart. At which point I started to panic… "Quick, phone the midwife!" When she arrived fifteen minutes later, she examined me to find I was already 8cm dilated and well into established labour.

The only way I could get comfortable was on the loo, as it seemed to relieve the pressure on my back and bum, and of course with the aid of gas and air. Doreen stayed with me the whole time and let me and my labour guide her. She suggested moving to the bedroom unless I wanted to give birth on the loo, so in between contractions I went, where she examined me again. At this point I was 9cm.

She called the second midwife and told her to drop everything and come quick. Once Kath arrived Doreen suggested breaking my waters as they were the only thing keeping this baby in. I was that high on gas and air I just slurred, "Yeah whatever." Once broken, I turned onto my side, which helped with the pains in my back, and had the urge to push immediately; I was amazed how you instinctively know what to do. After only fifteen minutes my daughter Lauren was born, weighing 8lb 2oz. It had been just four hours from my first contraction.

I cannot begin to describe how elated, tired, exhausted and relieved I felt. Wayne was literally speechless with pride and ecstatic at the arrival of his daughter. Lauren was passed straight to me to nurse. It felt so natural, just my new family and the midwives. A little while passed and Kath ran me a bath while Doreen cleaned up, then they both changed the bed sheets for me. I can't thank them enough for making my labour and birth such a wonderful experience.

My daughter is now almost two and such a contented child. She is so laid back and calm, everyone comments on it. I do believe it has a lot to do with such a relaxed birth in our home. It's no wonder I decided to have our second child at home. It took a little longer as Jay weighed eleven pounds. Needless to say I will definitely be having our next child at home too.

For me, the advantages of having a home birth far outweighed those of giving birth in hospital. Doreen came to the house for all my checks including regular check ups and blood tests, which brought us closer. Nothing was too much trouble – all I had to do if I had any worries was call her any time, day or night. Everything was provided for my labour; all I had to provide was me and my home. I would recommend home birth to anyone: it's a wonderful thing.

II

Partners' Perspectives

Mark's story

Fred, 2003

There's a picture on the stairs of our two children: Josie, aged 2 years and 364 days, and Fred, just under one day old. Josie's face is beaming, full of the joys that we're celebrating her birthday – well, technically it was the day before her birthday, but she didn't seem too concerned about those minor details! It had been quite a day for her: both sets of grandparents and her uncle had come to visit, she'd been given her first proper bicycle and, most importantly, she'd met her little brother for the first time. Fred, or 'Ped' as Josie preferred to call him at that point, looked every bit like Winston Churchill (complete with the V-sign), but cooched up so delicately in a tiny new-born babygrow, with his eyes squinting in the extremes of daylight, he was a joy to behold.

Whenever I see the picture, I'm reminded of that special day and the home birth that led to it. We had actually got together for three reasons: Fred's birth the day before, our wedding anniversary (the same day) and Josie's birthday the day after, but it was the opportunity for us all to be together, so soon after the birth, that made 17 August 2003 so completely memorable. From being three people and a bump two days before, we were now a proper, four-person family unit, and the opportunity to welcome Fred into this world, in the same surroundings that would become his home, couldn't have given him a more perfect start to his life.

The decision to have a home birth had, understandably, been driven by Hannah. Certainly, from giving birth to Josie, we'd

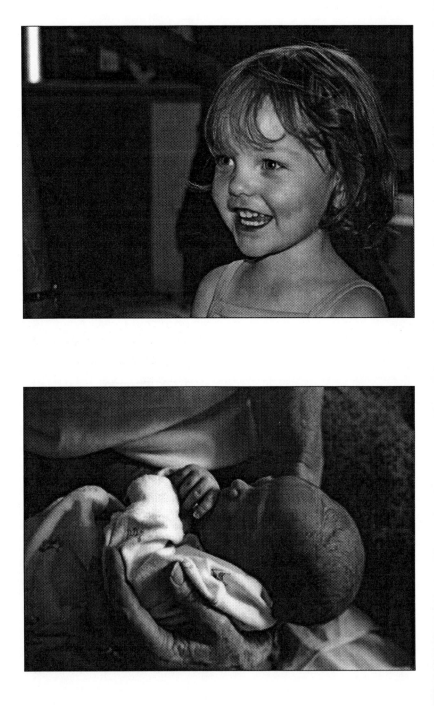

both realised that her body actually could push babies out (as flippant as that sounds, you never quite believe it until the head pops out!) and that, given a calm, relaxed environment, Hannah might not need so much pain medication. From my perspective, going into hospital the first time round felt like it slowed down Josie's birth; the more time Hannah could spend at home, the greater opportunity her body would have to 'do the right thing'. Of course, the fact that we lived only two miles from the hospital provided an important mental safety net, but ultimately, Fred's home birth felt like something we could achieve together.

Hannah went into labour during the Friday night, with my supportive response being to simply roll over and carry on sleeping! By early morning, I'd dutifully rung the midwife, Mandy, and told her that our boy was on his way, as well as assembling a makeshift bed in the downstairs kitchen from a futon mattress tastefully covered in a plastic sheet. The one thing I'd learnt from Josie's birth, and quite unlike the perspective of labour that you see on the TV, was that giving birth is (on the whole) a long, drawn out process. Rather than panicking and trying to do everything at once, I made sure I was there for Hannah and could steadily help her through each contraction.

The early hours of labour were interspersed with short walks around our neighbourhood, Hannah gripping my hand hard and occasionally stopping to make strange moaning sounds with her head rested against my chest. As bizarre as the sight of us must have looked, the walks really helped set a comfortable and assured pace through those early contractions – no rushing to get to level 10 on the tens machine, but a means of coping with the pain without getting too absorbed in it.

By this point Mandy had arrived, and later on in the day, two other midwives to take over her shift, as Fred's birth was clearly not going to be a 'three-hour wonder' like some other fortunate mothers seem to have. What surprised me the most about the midwives was how gentle and reassuring their presence was, most of the time simply letting Hannah and myself get on with things, but being there to answer questions and provide support and advice when needed. At times, they almost merged into our domestic existence – like when Mandy sat quietly in the front room filling out her notes, or when the two replacement midwives measured Hannah's dilation in between flicking through the pages of the *OK*, *Hello* and *Heat* magazines I'd bought from the Co-op earlier.

As time went on, Hannah tried to find the right place in our house to give birth. The futon construction I'd assembled in the kitchen had, not surprisingly, been ditched, and the use of our small bathroom felt slightly impractical, as there was barely room for us all to fit it. In the end, we relocated back into the master bedroom, but time had moved on to the point where a trip to hospital started to look increasingly inevitable. As with Josie's birth, Hannah's contractions had produced some dilation, but there were still a good few centimetres to go. As her waters hadn't broken, we were faced with the difficult decision of whether or not to break them – doing it would make the contractions more painful, but at the same time, it could aid the labour's development.

Siting on our bed, trying to work out what was best (by this time Hannah was guzzling the gas and air as if there was no tomorrow!) was certainly the toughest point for me in the whole process. Part of me was concerned for what Hannah had gone through and the potential pain the decision could lead to, the other part realised that breaking her waters could finally give the contractions the chance they needed to do their job. Unlike the 'difficult' decisions in hospital however, the discussion and conclusion we came to with the midwives' support felt calm, clear and informed. We decided to break the waters...

Suddenly things changed. After getting increasingly dizzy on gas and air, Hannah became focused, her breathing markedly different and her body clearly getting into the next phase of labour. Yet, at the same time, I remember the mood of the room becoming surprisingly relaxed. Hannah asked for a cup of tea, and so we all sat there sipping away as Fred slowly made his way. Even as Hannah began to push, we were still lounging around with our cups of tea, conversations jumping between stories in the magazines and the birth that was unfolding. It was a lovely and completely natural moment, although bloody painful I'm sure, but one where Hannah seemed in absolute control of what was happening, with the midwives ready to do their bit.

And so, at about 9:30pm that Saturday night, Fred Johnny Sawtell-Cousins was born, in the far corner of our bedroom, next to the radiator...

As the midwives got out their needle and thread, I carried Fred through to his bedroom. I watched as his face slowly turned from a bluish, 'just popped out into the real world' kind of colour to a peachy pink. Now and again he'd try to open his eyes, probably only to see a bright collection of incoherent blurs, but in a small way, it was our first connection as father and son. It was one of those few special moments in life you'll never forget – like when I walked into the maternity ward the day after Josie was born, or the day in February 1975 when I first met my younger brother, Johnny. Every time I see the photo of a one-day-old Fred at the top of our stairs, my mind is cast back to the exact feeling of holding him for the first time.

Sometimes, it's hard to believe that that little bundle I held in their bedroom is now the strapping young gentlemen, all of two and a bit years, that wanders around the house – chatting, playing with cars, or banging away on the synthesisers in my studio! Needless to say, Fred's Churchillian looks of old have been replaced by a curly set of locks and a rather cheeky smile, and Josie and Fred are both inseparable and the best of friends. Home birth, beyond all the benefits that it clearly offered Hannah, is one of the most wonderful ways to bring a child into the world, and I will treasure the time that Hannah, the midwives, Fred and I spent together on that beautiful August day.

Andy's story

Egan, 2002

From the very first moment that we became aware of our status as parents to be, or maybe an hour after seeing the fateful two pink lines, we were certain that the home birth route was the way we wanted to go. Having a good friend who had managed to have both of her children at home and always spoke of the experience with a very positive attitude was, I'm sure, a clinching factor in making this decision.

We were fortunate from the onset of this pregnancy to have a midwife who was supportive and realistic about home births and appeared excited at the prospect. I was surprised by the response, as I was expecting to have a bit of a battle on our hands in light of this being our first birth; we had made ready for such an occurrence. The pregnancy itself was uneventful, in fact I would go as far as to say pretty textbook. I made sure Mary ate well and we went to local NCT classes. Mary consulted a local homeopath who armed us with a pregnancy kit and, along with an auspicious shower curtain that had born witness to two previous home births and a vast assortment of old bedding and a beanbag, we were ready.

The wait for the impending pop was torture. As the due date came nearer, fears of what would happen if Mary had to go into hospital were continually at the back of my mind, mainly due to Mary's strong feeling that she did not wish to be in hospital. My biggest concern was 'How will she manage the pain ?' – especially as the experience of birth leads to realms which as a couple you have never met before. All these worries were proved unnecessary on B-day, which was about ten days after the due date (the wait had brought about a whole new set of unneeded worries, particularly the fear of induction).

I received a call from Mary at lunchtime to say that she thought she had started going into labour, so panic-stricken I raced through town in my car trying to get to grips with what the next 24 to 72 hours would have in store. All these weeks of preparation and at last, ten days late, we were ready for the off. Mary was on the phone when I came crashing into the house, red cape at the ready. Everything was calm and we eased into the process of timing contractions, started the TENS machine, and made a call to the midwife. She made a preliminary visit and asked us to call her again when we felt things were beginning to speed up.

I remember the constant phone calls from family and friends who were ringing to see if we had had the baby, and the shocked and horrified voices of people who spoke to Mary between contractions which confirmed to them that we were trying our best. The pain issue was managed very well with the TENS, twenty minutes of gas and air and a variety of homeopathic compresses. Things did speed up and approximately seven hours later we were blessed with a baby boy. Two hours after the birth we were left alone at home: the three of us, a bottle of bubbly and the cat.

I sometimes think the whole experience was so textbook it feels untrue. Mary managed the pain so well, the whole event ran so smoothly. When I tell people, they look at me like I'm a lunatic who doesn't know what he's talking about, particularly mothers who have had very different experiences. However, I remember very clearly the fun and laughs we had throughout that day. Our second son was also born at home some 23 months later, again a textbook delivery, just with much less of the unknown involved.

For another perspective on this experience, you can read Mary's story on p.127

Loz's story

Alex, 2005

I remember Ness telling me she was pregnant. She was supposed to be meditating that afternoon. I was trying to be quiet around the flat that we lived in at the time, but knew that I could go in the same room without disturbing her too much. I think I went in for a book and there she was, just sitting in the middle of the bed looking really coy. She told me to sit down and then blurted it all out. I was gobsmacked. We had talked about getting pregnant, and had actively made changes so that it was possible, but this was so soon it didn't seem real.

We talked a little about what it might mean, when it would happen (mid December), and how we felt. We agreed not to tell anyone until around twelve weeks which put us just after we were due to get married in late May. Then Ness realised she would be eight or nine weeks pregnant when we were due to get married and started to worry she might 'show'. There wasn't much we could do about it really other than tell the shop to leave a little room for movement in the dress. In the event, she didn't show and looked fantastic in her wedding dress. Somehow, nobody noticed she didn't drink any alcohol all day.

So to the birth story. We had agreed on a home birth, or rather Ness had suggested it as a possibility and I, never having thought about it before, agreed it sounded like a good idea. Neither of us is particularly fond of hospitals. I have quite a reputation for collapsing at the mere mention of a hypodermic needle and being over six feet tall it's something I try to avoid at all costs. I was still worried about how I would fare with all the blood and stuff being so squeamish, but decided to put it out of my mind and deal with it on the day. Both of us are 'water babies' too so we also agreed that we would research a water birth and see whether it would be feasible to do at home.

At our 16-week appointment with our community midwife, Julie, we broached the home birth subject with trepidation. We had heard that midwives aren't particularly fond of home births but for what reason, and from what source the information came, we weren't sure. Julie was firm and quick. It wasn't something we could discuss with her until the 37-week check-up. Only then would she know if Ness's iron levels and blood pressure would be on the home birth bandwagon too. To be honest she seemed rather distant at that moment. Both Ness and I have reconciled ourselves with her approach – for a midwife to give false hope very early on must be quite hard to deal with later – but for us we would have preferred to take that risk and talk about it anyway.

We had also decided that we wanted to take antenatal classes much earlier than the NHS provided classes so we booked ourselves onto a hypnobirthing course. Hypnobirthing teaches you essentially two things. Firstly, how to breathe during labour, both during and between contractions and for the pushing itself. Secondly, you are taught to interpret the whole experience of birth in a less clinical, more natural way. As women have been giving birth since the beginning, and we as a society have only medicalised birth in the last fifty years, then clearly hospital shouldn't be the presumptive choice. With a renewed vigour for breathing, and a completely different mindset on birth itself we both felt much more confident that we would not only survive the experience, but look back at it in a positive light too.

Our well-researched birthing pool turned up, and we set about moving furniture to create a comfortable environment in which Ness could experience labour and the birth of our baby.

We had an appointment with our osteopath for some cranio-sacral work on the Monday following the due date, just in case the baby didn't arrive on time on the Sunday. Sunday came and went and at 9am on Monday Ness was lying down on the table being worked on by Imogen. Cheerily going about her business, Imogen informed Ness that her contractions would begin around 10:30 that morning. Back home, laughing over a cup of tea and toast, Ness had her first contraction. It was 10:30am.

They came sporadically through the day, twenty minutes apart, fifteen, eight, then ten and back up to twenty. We decided to go to bed around midnight to give ourselves some rest for what was to come. We hadn't even let our heads hit the pillow when at half past midnight they suddenly started to come stronger and more frequently. The small hours of the morning for Ness were spent watching *The West Wing* on DVD downstairs and alternating from chair to exercise ball to standing. I slept for a few hours on the sofa.

We'd attached the TENS machine already and were starting to get used to how it worked. It was a little tricky as Ness couldn't speak during contractions so we'd have to liaise between goes to get the settings right. At the same time we used some Shiatsu pressure points at the base of Ness's back to relieve pain. These were unfortunately at the same place as the TENS pads so my thumbs started to go to sleep after a few hours. Obviously I kept my mouth firmly closed about this seemingly insignificant 'discomfort' I was experiencing. This was not a competition!

We called our midwife around 8am, and she came over an hour later to check Ness over. After popping out for supplies, she came back at 10:30am to stay. We were cheerily told at this point that Ness was 5cm dilated and this could all be done by mid to late afternoon.

Around midday we decided to fill the pool. The contractions by now were strong and clearly spaced apart by three minutes or so. The pool took much longer to fill than I expected as we (apparently) have a small water tank, so about an hour and a half later it was ready to use. The birthing pool made a big difference to Ness in terms of natural pain relief. Instantly she was in a better place, more relaxed and able to regroup and carry on. My role at this point was to keep an eye on the temperature of the pool and carry buckets of hot water between the kitchen and the study.

By 4:30 Ness was fully dilated. Labour had started around sixteen hours previously. This pushing phase involved Ness being in the pool, walking around the house, sitting on the floor and climbing the stairs to move around. An hour and a half later Ness was still pushing hard and we were getting a little concerned that nothing was happening. The midwife was routinely checking baby's heartbeat to make sure everything was still okay. Ness was becoming a little dispirited too and to give her a lift the midwife got hold of her hand and placed it on the crown of the baby's head. Ness was inspired and carried on for another half an hour with even more effort than before.

At 7pm, though, the midwife had to make a call. We had openly discussed going to hospital in the event that we couldn't deliver at home. It was even on the birth plan in language that both Ness and I agreed with: we go to hospital if a medical reason dictates just that.

The ambulance was called. Ness continued to have contractions while we waited and I dealt with a small but worrisome leak our pool appeared to have sprung (turned out to be the drainage plug not quite seated properly).

Once in the hospital our community midwife, Julie, handed over to the hospital midwives so that our history and needs were explained fully. This was really important to both of us. Ness was already starting to worry about what was happening to her and that we didn't really understand what was going on. We persisted in asking what the doctor was doing and why, and what was going to happen. The hospital put Ness on a dose of Syntocinon to regulate and force the contractions. Once this had kicked in then they could decide how to go forward in terms of delivery. The contractions were really strong and Ness agreed to start using gas and air to help. This seemed to reduce the acuity of the pain, but gave her a slightly spacey feel.

After an hour or so the doctor came in and assessed the position of the baby's head (transverse – which explains why nothing was moving at home). Things moved very quickly and we felt a little disregarded at this stage. After pushing for an answer we realised that the doctor was going to use Neville Barnes forceps following an episiotomy. A local anaesthetic helped to reduce the sting of the incision, but Ness was still in a great deal of pain. The use of the forceps also caused immense pain for Ness, but once they were in the delivery of Alex was fairly quick, as was the delivery of the placenta. All happened in the space of four or five contractions: a little baby boy weighing 7lb 10oz.

After the delivery the doctor had to stitch the episiotomy which was apparently much more painful than anything that had happened previously, including the delivery. Ness was cleaned up (so much blood it's truly a miracle I stayed standing), and Alex was put in a wheeled crib next to the bed.

The midwives at the hospital on the labour suite were fantastic and, although they could have done more to explain what was happening, cared for Ness's every need while she was in there.

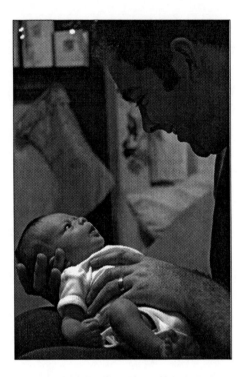

Six weeks on, Ness and baby Alex are doing just fine. We are a little concerned that the Syntocinon may be the cause of Alex being colicky, but it'll pass. The main thing is he's alert and putting on weight. We were a little upset that Alex wasn't born at home, but there's always next time!

For another perspective on this experience, you can read Ness's story on p.171

Paul's stories

Max, 2002

Tracy had two children from a previous marriage while I had none. Both of her children had been born at the City Hospital, Nottingham and she had had fairly easy labours without complications. When we found out we were expecting our first child it came as a bit of a shock but a very nice one. Once we got over the fact that we were pregnant we had to make all sorts of decisions. Firstly, whether we should have the tests recommended for mothers over 35 years of age at the time of the birth. With all the decisions we had to make, discussing where to give birth didn't really feature at first.

Tracy came home one day after visiting the midwife saying she had discussed the possibility of home birth. She also talked to a neighbour who had given birth at home. Although Tracy was really keen on the idea I was a bit more nervous. I didn't know what to expect or what to do, whereas she had previous experience! Over the coming months we talked about it on several occasions. Although it didn't stop my worries, she was confident that this was what she wanted so I went with it, albeit it with reservations.

On a visit to the midwife towards the end of the pregnancy she gave us a list of items to shop for and recommended Wilko's for the plastic ground sheet. We had to have sheets, towels, sanitary towels, a bucket, baby clothes and nappies. I got on really well with the midwife and often enjoyed some banter; I hoped she would be on duty when the time came. She constantly assured me that a home birth is a lovely experience and nothing to worry about.

D-Day. I was out walking the dogs when Tracy phoned me to say that she thought her waters had broken after getting out of the bath. I came straight home. Tracy had already phoned the midwife to report the progress, and the midwife said she would call within half an hour. No contractions had started. Unfortunately our midwife was not on duty, but we need not have worried, the on-call midwife was lovely.

Jackie arrived at the house and inspected Tracy to give her opinion. The cervix was 3cm dilated but no contractions were apparent. We could be in for a long night! She left telling us to call her if things started to happen and that she would let the second midwife know she would probably be called out in the early hours. We sat at home with anticipation waiting for the contractions. Within half an hour of Jackie leaving they started. She had just got home and changed when the call came to come straight back.

By the time Jackie arrived, Tracy's contractions were progressing rapidly and it was all systems go. The sheet was on the floor and she was bent over a dining chair. We had a Faith Hill CD on and I got myself a glass of wine. There were so many emotions in the room it was really hard to comprehend what was shortly going to happen. Jackie took control from the minute she walked through the door and was reassuring and comforting to Tracy. She immediately contacted the second midwife as it was apparent the birth would be very soon.

Max was born around 11pm. Maria, the second midwife, took hold of him and checked him over while Jackie concentrated on Tracy, monitoring the delivery of the placenta and checking that she was okay. Max looked so small. He was handed back to Tracy after a few minutes and we both had a lovely little cuddle with him and checked him out, his nose, his eyes, his ears, his hands, everything. He was perfect. I called my mum to let her know she had a new grandson and Tracy called her mum too.

After a couple of hours Jackie left and advised us to try and get some sleep. We later found out that it had been her first home delivery. The weirdest thing was to have this little chap to carry upstairs in his Moses basket and then try to sleep.

The whole experience was extremely comfortable for me though I was apprehensive throughout. Jackie and Maria were both professional, polite and very respectful. I had read that bonding is more effective with a home delivery – I hadn't experienced a hospital birth to compare it to, but it was just lovely to see my baby and wife look so content. I would happily have another home birth.

Martha, 2005

Hey ho, she's pregnant again!

No doubt that a home birth would be the way to go. The pregnancy was relatively simple, though Tracy had a few problems at about seven months which would have put a spanner in the works had they been proven. Once again we had the same community midwife throughout the pregnancy. She had been disappointed that she wasn't on duty for Max's birth and was determined not to miss out on this one. Once again she sent me shopping for the items needed. By this time decorators sheets were very popular in our household.

Tracy had a hindwater tear at around 39 weeks but nothing happened. We contacted the midwife who came promptly and checked her out. For the next 36 hours there were midwives in and out of the house checking that all was well. At this stage we were concerned that if nothing happened contraction-wise we would have to go to hospital for the delivery.

Finally, two days later at 2am the contractions started. Tracy woke me and asked me to call the midwife straight away as she lived a fair distance. It was going to be our community midwife this time! My sister came to collect the older children as they didn't want to be present.

Contractions came thick and fast and for a moment I thought I would be delivering our child, but Elaine made it. She didn't have time even to have a drink; she was involved very quickly and within fifteen to twenty minutes of her arrival, baby Martha was born. Tracy delivered in the same position that she had for Max – over the dining chair in the living room.

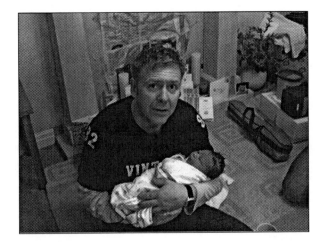

After the birth of Max I had read that skin contact creates a bonding with your child so I took my T-shirt off and cuddled her. Elaine checked Tracy out and everything seemed okay. The whole experience again for me was lovely. An absolutely wonderful experience for both Tracy and myself.

For another perspective on this experience, you can read Tracy's story on p.27

Tom's stories

Rosie, 2004

When we found out Aby was pregnant, we were in no doubt that we would plan a home birth. Partly this was because we'd had a previous pregnancy which miscarried, so a lot of our thinking had been done already. But even before that, we had talked through the process of birth (as Aby was a student midwife, the subject was often discussed) and realised we were both naturally inclined to the idea of labour and birth at home.

It's easy to see where the impetus came from for Aby – her younger brother was born at home and her mother was involved for years with the NCT – but I'm less sure what informed my decision. My brother, my sister and I were all born in hospital and I didn't have experience of anyone close to me giving birth at home until my brother's wife in the summer of 2000. Aby popped in with a bunch of flowers to wish her well on her due date and accidentally became the baby's first visitor! Her description of the cosy informality of the scene just a couple of hours after the birth made it seem very warm, domestic and natural.

Another brick in the wall was reading Ina May Gaskin's book *Spiritual Midwifery*. This 1970s classic is full of hippy couples describing effusively how "strong" their births were and how they got "really high on the vibes". It has some of the most remarkable beards and kaftans I've ever seen. But behind the flower power aesthetic, it shows how couples can deliver their babies in the same spirit of love and warmth in which they were conceived.

This reinforced my own strong sense that, as mammals, our natural reaction to labour is to find somewhere safe, secure and comfortable, keep strangers at bay and just get on with things. Given that I'd always felt a bit anxious in hospitals, unsure of what I should be doing and put off by the smell of disinfectant, I knew that *I* would feel more comfortable at home. I could thoroughly understand the appeal to Aby, who actually had to get down to the business of giving birth.

Above all this, I was inspired by Aby's growing sense as she studied that midwifery is different from other branches of medicine (you could even say it's *not* a branch of medicine) in that generally no-one involved is ill. Why is it necessary to be in hospital if mother and baby are only doing something natural? Reading her midwifery journals, it seemed that hospital birth was too often subject to over-cautious interventions, and I became aware of the way in which one intervention leads to another: an epidural can slow contractions, which may then be encouraged with a hormone drip; or it can hamper the action of the pelvic floor muscles and three hours later out come the forceps.

We opted for a home birth, united in our belief that it would provide the best experience for all concerned. Aby would feel secure and relaxed in our own home, so wouldn't need all the pain relief options provided in hospital. We would have low lighting and comfy cushions, the birth ball would be out and we would have access to all the goodies with which we had stocked the fridge. Once Aby reached 5cm dilated, she would climb into the birth pool we had hired and the last stages of labour would happen in our kitchen with just me and Aby, her mum and the attendant midwives to welcome our new baby into the world. In the end, though, things didn't happen quite like that.

On a Tuesday morning a week after due date, I was shaken awake by Aby to be informed that her waters had broken. The soggy mess on her half of the bedsheet confirmed this, and justified our having spent a week sleeping with a pad under the sheet. I got up excitedly, but she wasn't experiencing any contractions so, at my usual time I headed off for work. I knew that it might take days for contractions to start and didn't want to waste my paternity leave before it was needed. By lunchtime, though, I realised my mind wasn't on work and when my MD told me in no uncertain terms to clear off home to my wife, I took him at his word.

It turned out I *was* needed at home, not because there was any sign of contractions starting but because there wasn't: Aby was increasingly anxious about the prospect of induction and needed me alongside for reassurance. It didn't help that the community midwife on duty (not our own but another member of the team) immediately talked about having to whip Aby into hospital for monitoring within 24 hours of her waters breaking due to the risk of infection. This didn't fit with our idea of natural childbirth.

Aby quickly got in touch with the midwife who had volunteered to be first on call for her – a friend from her time spent on placement. She told us that the hospital's protocol actually specified monitoring within 48 hours of membrane rupture and induction within 72 hours. This talk of protocols got us thinking, and we swiftly went online to look for the NICE guidelines (the national recommendations which inform hospitals' own practice). Here it was stated that induction should begin within 96 hours, which we seized on with relief. This gave us a bit more time, and grounds for putting up a fight if pressure was put on us to go for an early induction.

Still, we were relieved when, at 1am on the Thursday, less than 48 hours after her waters broke, Aby began feeling regular contractions. We got up excitedly, lit candles in the bedroom and I went to find a pack of cards, thinking that gin rummy might while the hours away. A very peaceful scene, then, until about 3am when I started to feel decidedly peculiar. My stomach was churning and I felt dizzy. Perhaps I was feeling nervous about the birth, I thought, or about the suddenly imminent reality of being a father. But six hours later, after endless bouts of vomiting and diarrhoea, I recognised that my dodgy ham sandwiches of the previous evening had been more to blame. I felt tired, sorry for myself, and utterly useless as a birth partner for Aby at the time when she needed me most.

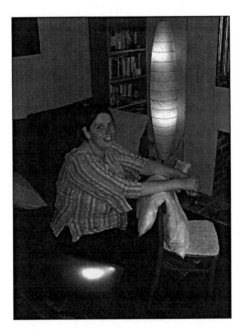

Fortunately, Aby was doing fine on her own terms. Standing for every contraction, she was swaying and moaning gently through the pain before sitting again to write in her diary or continue chatting to her mum, who had joined us at about 5am to help put the birth pool up and compensate for my state of weak-kneed nausea. With Corinne there and Aby coping well, I gratefully accepted the suggestion that I get some sleep. A few hours later I felt much more on form, and came downstairs to find the scene very little changed.

In fact, little changed for the rest of the day. Contractions continued to arrive every ten minutes or so, at times clustering closer together before fading off again. For every one Aby was up on her feet and swaying, with me applying increasing pressure to her lower back and, through the later hours, with the gas-and-air nozzle firmly between her teeth.

By 5am on Friday, we were all tired. Aby hadn't eaten much and internals still showed that dilation hadn't gone past 3-4cm and the baby was still high up the birth canal. Given that the last exam had suggested the baby might be facing the wrong way, we wondered whether all those hours of contractions had been spent turning the baby round. Now, with Aby tired and her contractions fading, we decided it was worth going to hospital to see if a Syntocinon drip could give the extra boost needed to get this baby out. We piled into the car – me, Aby, Corinne, midwife, gas tank and all – and drove the few minutes to the maternity ward.

The hospital was very different from our cosy living room. We'd been cocooned in a world of our own for 24 hours, with curtains closed, lights low and Van Morrison on the stereo. Now the lights were bright and there were people everywhere. Looking back I'm not surprised that the contractions virtually disappeared when we got into the hospital. Though everyone was very friendly and helpful, the atmosphere was so different. While waiting for everything to be set up for the induction, I sat around feeling a bit like a spare part and talking in weary monosyllables to Aby and Corinne.

The mood changed, though, when the Syntocinon began to kick in and the contractions were coming faster and stronger than ever. Now Aby was up on her feet again, and my mother-in-law and I were back in supportive mode – Corinne at Aby's head with words of encouragement and sips of water, me standing behind Aby to apply near-constant pressure on her lower back. I hardly noticed the midwives: I think they could see that we'd developed a strong sense of teamwork through all that time labouring at home and there wasn't much they needed to do. Every ten minutes or so they adjusted the belt holding the CTG monitor, checked the baby's vital signs and made sure the IV lines for the Syntocinon and antibiotics were doing their job. Then they left us to it.

In the end, the last stage was quick. Aby had a textbook emotional five minutes at transition, which her mum talked her through wonderfully, then there were 45 minutes of pushing. She squatted for this and I was finally let off lumbar duty. I moved down to the business end and, as the midwives scrambled around on the floor to get low enough to catch, I saw my baby crowning.

I was amazed that Aby could open up that much, and stunned to actually see my baby's head – a real, grey-pink, hairy baby's head. But more than anything I was so, so proud of this resourceful woman, my wife, who had been on her feet for most of 36 hours, had stuck to her convictions about pain relief and, despite the tubes in both arms, the bulky CTG belt and the punishing intensity of hormone-induced contractions, had achieved the active birth she wanted.

The midwives respected our birth plan to the very last. So, after the anxiety I felt on seeing our floppy grey bundle of baby had turned to relief as she began crying and gradually turning pink, I was handed my child to discover for myself what kind of being we'd created. I was staggered to discover it was a girl, though I think I'd have been equally astonished if it had been a boy: the very fact of her having a gender made her so much

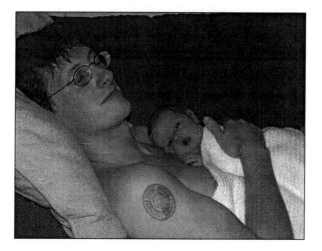

more a real, living human being. I was pleased, too, knowing that Aby had secretly been wanting a girl for all of nine months of pregnancy.

Keeping my discovery to myself, I handed Rosie over without a word and was rewarded by Aby's own effusive reaction to having a daughter.

Bede, 2005

From early in our relationship, Aby and I had agreed that if we were going to have children together we'd want to have several. Soon after Rosie was born we decided not to plan ongoing contraception, so it was no great surprise when, with Rosie seven months old, we found out we were expecting again.

Our desire to go for a home birth was no less fervent than it had been the first time round. The experience of labouring at home had been wholly positive, food poisoning aside, and we were keen to see if we could go the whole distance this time. We had learned some lessons from Rosie's birth – particularly for me the importance of trying to get food into Aby during labour to keep her energy levels high – and were optimistic about a second attempt. After all, labours are generally shorter with a second baby so it probably wouldn't be another 35-hour marathon.

An important difference was that we now had Rosie to think about, but this only seemed like another good reason to be at home. Just as a home birth allows the father to spend more of those vital first few days with a new baby, it would mean that Rosie would get to meet her new brother or sister early on and in her own home; mummy wouldn't be disappearing for days before arriving back in the house with an interloper.

In many ways, this second pregnancy felt less intense than the first. For a start, both Aby and I were too busy looking after Rosie to spend time daydreaming about our new baby or endlessly repeating our shortlist of acceptable names. Neither were we going to the NCT antenatal classes which had been so useful (for me at least) before Rosie's birth.

At about 37 weeks, it suddenly struck home that we really were having another baby and, moreover, that between now and being a father of two I would have to do my best again to support Aby through labour. At this realisation, I spent a few days anxiously trying to remember everything we'd learned in the NCT classes about useful positions, massage in labour and how to help Aby with her breathing. The pressure on me felt greater this time because Corinne wasn't going to be there to help – we had agreed that this time her role as grandmother would be to look after Rosie for as long as was needed while Aby was in labour.

At news of this Aby's twin sister leapt to fill the gap. It wasn't fair, she said, that Aby as a student midwife had been present at so many births and she hadn't seen any except her own son's! Please, please, please could she be there?

I was quite relaxed about the idea, which surprised even me. When Verity had asked to attend Rosie's birth I had been dead set against it. Being partner to an identical twin leads to a certain amount of wrangling over the pecking order of affection, and it's hard to feel completely secure of your position next to someone who has been your partner's closest friend and confidante their whole life.

Now, though, things felt very different. The experience of shared parenting had cemented mine and Aby's relationship more than I ever expected, and I didn't experience Verity as a threat any more. In the end it was Aby who decided she would rather it was just the two of us.

Aside from this, our birth plan had changed very little. We had bought rather than hired a birth pool (and were amused that our giant inflatable paddling pool was festooned with tropical fish – I kept threatening to don a hula skirt for the labour) and booked a TENS machine, but otherwise we were simply hoping to have now the birth we had planned 15 months earlier.

At one day before due date, it suddenly looked as if that might be an unlikely prospect. At a routine doctor's appointment, Aby was told that the doctor thought the baby might be breech, and we rushed to hospital for a scan which confirmed the suspicion. Fortunately, we opted for an external cephalic version, and the midwife and Aby between them managed to get the baby to turn and stay turned.

A few days later, it was Aby's waters breaking that again signalled the start of proceedings. This time, it was on a Sunday evening while she was on the phone to a friend, which was the cause of some hilarity. I remember being much less nervous at this point than the previous time – I felt only a matter-of-fact sense of being pleased to get on with the labour and meet our new baby.

Contractions started fairly quickly, but it wasn't until 10.00 the next morning, when they were coming routinely every ten minutes and seeming as if they meant business, that Aby settled and began to enjoy the labour. We played Trivial Pursuit and she sucked ice lollies between contractions. It felt like a very special time, just the two of us, and I was amazed by how, though the contractions were coming on strong, as soon as each was done, Aby was right back on form, laughing and getting on with the game.

It was after we ran out of lollies that Verity appeared on the scene after all. Aby called her desperately to commission a supermarket trip and she arrived with emergency supplies at just the most useful point, when Aby was approaching transition and the midwife had still not turned up. I think just having another woman around made a difference to Aby, and we quickly suggested Verity should stay. She promised to be inconspicuous and volunteered to take photos, which was a great idea: without her there I certainly wouldn't have been free to get any pictures.

A minute or two later the midwife arrived, and from then on things progressed very quickly. As soon as she had done an internal exam and pronounced that Aby could get in the pool, we dashed into the kitchen and Aby clambered in. This furnished the comedy moment of the day, as Aby forgot to switch off the TENS machine before thrusting the electrodes into my hands. I felt the judder of electric shocks she'd hardly been noticing, and as I pulled the sticky pads off one hand they just stuck to the other!

Very quickly after getting in the pool, Aby said she could feel the baby coming and began to get worried that everything was happening too quickly, especially as the midwife was still unpacking her bag. She was on all fours at this point, so I suggested she move to a more laid-down position to slow things up a bit. I moved behind her and she sat back against me and gratefully accepted the drink Verity offered. Then, as I remember, it, she very calmly delivered the baby's head.

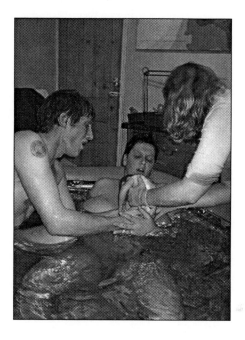

The next few minutes were surreal. We could see the baby's head between Aby's legs and I remember touching it and finding the ears, trying to work out which way it was facing. Sue – the midwife – told me I'd need to turn the baby as the body was delivered but I wasn't really taking in her instructions. In the end, I just helped the baby move the way it seemed naturally to be going and all in one big slither I held my baby son in my hands. This time I was prepared for how wet and grey and floppy he would be, and just lifted him up onto Aby's chest to get his breath and discover the world slowly.

I was elated to be so involved at this point, and overjoyed that the birth had gone smoothly. Aby and I looked at each other and cried, the baby fed a little and cried, Aby's mum came into the room and cried – it was great! When Rosie came in she signed 'Baby' a few times then just stood by the pool sucking her thumb and taking it all in. Perhaps she was wondering why mummy and daddy were having a bath in the kitchen.

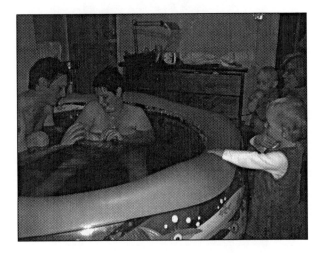

As we sat with new and extended family in the living room drinking champagne, I felt strongly all the benefits of being at home. We were warm and snug in our own space, and already settling into the patterns of being a family of four.

For another perspective on this experience, you can read Aby's story on p.61

Jon's story

Dan, 2004

After Katie, our first, turned out to be breech and was born by planned caesarean section, Karen was decidedly edgy and panicky as she wanted a home birth. I stayed calm.

When Dan was due, Karen got irritated by the midwives over the home birth issue, and again, I had to stay calm. Until Karen contacted Lis, an independent midwife (at 39 weeks!). Her serenity immediately calmed Karen and left me suddenly without that responsibility and without the control I had had. That is when I realised how much of a gooseberry I was going to be in all of this…

So, how to be the proverbial gooseberry at the party? Whatever they say about a man's role in labour, there was very little that I could do. My first task was to ring the grandparents at 7am and notify them that "Something's happening" then drop off our two-year-old daughter Katie at nursery. Mainly I supplied herbal tea at half-hourly intervals to the midwives around the birth pool and kept the Santana CD on permanent play. (Changing it to Enya when I got fed up of 'Black Magic Woman' on the third rendition was not a welcome move!) All Karen wanted was the occasional "Hello" to which she grunted approval and fell back to sleep.

So I did the washing: I managed three loads of laundry! I cleaned the kitchen and read the *New Scientist* with my feet up in the living room. It was a glorious February day, the birth pool was keeping the house steamed up like a sauna and I was keeping the doors and windows open and the neighbours up to date on progress. I had no significant involvement with proceedings until one in the morning, when the call came to get in the pool and stop Karen drowning... at which point my pausing to take my heavyweight jeans off (to give more movement, honestly!) was misconstrued as being neat and tidy.

Dan emerged, greyish and plump, and very obviously a boy – which surprised me because until that point I think I'd expected another girl. He was quiet and calm, quite unlike his sister who was demanding and noisy from the off. Can't say that of him any more.

As for the third stage of labour, I had nothing to do with it except to go and get the chips, and the onerous task of putting away the birth pool...

For another perspective on this experience, you can read Karen's story on p.191

Phill's story

Luke, 2005

My wife, Sarah, tells me the hospital birth of our first son, Joseph, in December 2003 was 'very easy' compared to what she was prepared for. I will never know how difficult it was; all I can say is that it was great experience for us both, the only down side being that I felt like a bit of a spare part.

When Sarah suggested we should have our second baby at home I did not hesitate to say yes. I don't like hospitals, I find them claustrophobic and would rather stay away, so the thought of a birth like Joseph's but in the comfort of our own home was ideal. The community midwives reassured us that this was a great way to have our second child and so we were even more positive about the prospect.

Our home is really comfortable and we enjoy living there so I couldn't think of a better place to have our baby: you know where everything is and after the birth people can come and go as they please and help themselves to drinks and snacks. I have always felt that if there were any complications we wouldn't think twice about having the birth at hospital, but we would want Sarah to be able to come home as soon as possible.

I read some information on home birth and questioned the midwives, mainly about things like what would happen if they didn't get there in time – their reply being that while this is very rare, if it did happen they would talk me through things on the phone until someone did get there.

Sarah did most of the preparation of items needed for the birth, but she took me through where everything was and we made sure that I knew where all the relevant phone numbers for the hospital were. I would say that there was a lot less preparation than for our hospital birth, possibly because it was second time round so we were more relaxed, and probably because we were in the comfort of our own home and more familiar with the surroundings.

Towards the end of Sarah's pregnancy we were on tenterhooks as Joseph had arrived three weeks early and we were expecting this baby to do similar. When Sarah did go into labour (at two days overdue!) things happened very quickly, but we were both calm and collected. I think as the dad you are always going to be a bit of a 'gopher' because the mum is the one in control. Saying that, when we had Joseph at hospital the midwives did all of the delivery and I just reassured Sarah. When he was born I cut the cord, but I did feel like a bit of a spare part. We knew none of the delivery team and, while they were a great team, it was fairly impersonal.

The whole environment at home is less clinical, bar the bag of delivery equipment, and I knew most (and Sarah had met all) of the midwives. We really liked all of them and in particular Jackie, who was the one I knew best. She made the whole experience throughout the pregnancy interesting and something to be excited about, not scared.

At home for Luke's birth I knew where everything was and relished the opportunity to be more involved. Only one midwife arrived in time for the birth, which I was secretly chuffed about as she allowed me to assist with the delivery of Luke, lifting him onto Sarah, as well as cutting his cord, after only 1 hour and 45 minutes of labour. Naturally when Luke was born I felt that indescribable feeling of complete elation and pride that stays with you forever. I think it really helped that Jackie was the midwife who delivered Luke – she really got me involved, even giving me a lesson on the placenta (before we fried it up for breakfast… only joking!).

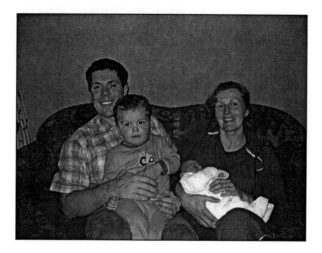

After our hospital birth I had to leave at about 8pm and went home to a house that was upside down. Joseph was three weeks early and we had been plastering a wall the day before so that was all still to clean up. While I was high as a kite, I then did not see Joseph for another 18 hours – the longest we've ever been apart! With Luke I don't think he left my sight for the first two days. I rang all our family and friends and everything just revolved around the comfort of our home.

Sarah has been brilliant through both labours and I think I dare say she 'takes it in her stride'. Both times she needed no pain relief and, especially with Luke, she was completely in control and showed no signs of panic or pain. That was always my biggest concern: that she would suffer a long drawn-out labour; so I am just very grateful for the way things went. I don't know how Sarah compares with other mothers but from the stories we have heard from friends I think we both realise that she is one of the lucky ones in labour and we are just really grateful for that.

As with Joseph's birth the experience was truly unforgettable and thankfully Sarah shared the same sentiments. In her usual way, she was up and about three hours after giving birth – what a star!

For another perspective on this experience, you can read Sarah's story on p.99

Robin's stories

Merrin, 2002

My wife, Kris, had borne two children at home prior to my two pests and to be honest she was happier about doing it again than I was. Experience I suppose. As a twenty-six-year-old whose only experience of child birth was when Pregnant Woman gives birth on a hijacked aeroplane or sinking oil rig (see disaster films of the 1970s), it seemed a given that the place to give birth is in a hospital. On the other hand, having been inside a hospital a few times I am not sure I would want to give birth there. My visits tended to be fairly stressful and, despite the assurances of *Casualty* and *Holby City*, hand washing doesn't appear to be a strong point.

My now four-year-old daughter was born first, in the flat we had at the time. I was called home from work in a hurry (missing my congratulatory pint at a local pub) and for two hours I walked my girlfriend round the block until this became uncomfortable. The on-call midwife was summoned and Kris got in the bath. At this point I was unhelpfully engaged in reading *Lord of the Rings*; I haven't yet lived this down and probably never will. Once the midwife arrived I sprang into action, putting the kettle on.

The midwife, who was the daughter of a friend of my dad's, assisted Kris into a number of positions while I hovered in the background feeling a bit shaky. It seemed as if everyone had done it before and I was waiting to see how it was done before I could have a go. I learned from my dawdlings and was much better next time.

The second midwife was due to arrive but hadn't when Merrin was born on our bedroom floor. I cut the cord. The second midwife phoned us as the placenta emerged – I was on my way to Kris and the midwife was on her way to speak to the second midwife.

Gabriel, 2004

I was much better prepared the second time and managed to make myself useful: lots of back rubbing and general encouragement. My son was born at home while the older boys slept and my little girl had gone to Grandma's.

There was no time for gas and air which I was told was available (but not to me) when the (different but very nice) midwife arrived. Her chum managed to arrive prior to the birth this time. Very soon, Gabriel was born and clothed: a squashed and washed-up beetroot in a blue suit with a dog on it.

Giving birth doesn't require a lot of space and the midwives will bring all the stuff they need. It can be surprisingly quick and being at home makes the whole thing less of a bother. I cannot imagine a hasty drive or an ambulance to hospital, the too-bright lights, the smells. Impersonality is just a curtains-draw away. It seems a shame to me to have to tag on such a misused word as 'Natural' (note the capital) to 'birth', which is arguably the most natural thing in nature.

For another perspective on this experience, you can read Kris's story on p.203

Ameet's story

Rohan, 2005

Getting ready for Rohan was a big task. Confident that home birth would be best for us, the only thing we needed was a home! Outpriced or under-earning – whichever way you want to look at it, we were moving.

Our new flat falling through three months before our due date wasn't ideal but it allowed us to rethink our lifestyle choices. We opted for a big upheaval (apparently this happens quite a lot before a baby comes) and if everything went to plan we'd move into a new city and have the baby at home. So we bought the first house we saw on Hannah's third day trip (ever) to Nottingham. Six weeks later we'd moved in and four weeks later baby was due.

Due to our living circumstances we were never sure that we would be able to go for the home birth we wanted, and only when we arrived and the sale of our house had gone through did we know that it would be possible. It was the option we felt happiest with: Hannah would be more relaxed at home and so the delivery would be shorter and easier as a result. As she was about to let go in a way she had never done before, she was going have to be more relaxed and grounded than ever.

I also felt that the midwives would be more sensitive towards our needs in our home than they would be on a busy hospital ward. What with all kinds of horror stories we had heard about rising and unusual rates of Caesarean sections, MRSA scares and so on, I felt if things got difficult we would be completely in the doctors' hands and I guess I didn't trust them that much.

After all, they were turning this natural beautiful process of Mother Nature's into a masculine process with various forceps and gadgets: basically boys with their toys. It just didn't feel right. I figured if we really needed a doctor we'd only be ten minutes away.

The baby was a week late by the time Hannah and I decided to go to the cinema, a sort of last date before the baby arrived. We were back and in bed by 12:30am. At 1:30 I heard a few shufflings and Hannah going to and back from the loo. Half asleep, I asked her if she was okay and she told me that she had diarrhoea and some contractions. Although she wasn't sure if this was actually it, for some reason I knew straight away that it was.

The week before, with my back done in by the house move and other emotions, I had gone to see an osteopath, a nice man who sorted my back out and happened to be a recent first-time father. He told me two things that really stayed with me. Firstly, that his wife's labour was preceded by diarrhoea, and secondly something else, very beautiful, which I'll share later in this birth story. Anyway, I knew it had begun. I knew that after we had been through this process, life would never be the same. Very soon there would be a little person to fill all those babygrows in the drawer.

With the diarrhoea came waves of what could only be contractions. I started to time them – only four minutes apart. I had thought they were quite close. I wanted to be near Hannah and support her while the contractions were happening and I tried to figure out how I was going to get the room and everything else ready.

I had a great faith that Hannah could get through each one and to help her we would use sound. We had already thought of some different methods we might be able to use to help ease the pain: sound, breathing and positions. I thought I would let her lead the way. Quite quickly I saw that the sound 'Maaa' in a low-pitched voice was giving her something to focus on and helping her to have long out breaths. I knew this would help her to let go into each contraction. 'Ma', meaning 'mother' in so many languages, was a sound to invoke Mother Nature to do her stuff. At the very least I also knew that making low-pitched sounds would help Hannah's lower regions to relax and let go, as well as keeping the baby relaxed.

In between contractions I was busy setting out mats, getting birthing balls, snacks, lighting, birth plans out, etc. On calling the midwife she said that Hannah had the signs of early labour. Mentally I was setting myself up for a long labour. How long, it was impossible to know.

Hannah had been looking forward to getting in the bath and once she was in the contractions seemed to change to a more manageable feeling. She seemed fine so I went along my business; even if I couldn't get to her for the contraction I made the 'Maa' sound just to let her know that I wasn't far away and to remind her that the contraction would end by the end of the sound.

In hindsight it was great to have something to do. I felt I was empowered to help with Hannah's pain. I had read in so many books that men feel helpless. I remember a sense that labour was sort of really human and hadn't changed since the dawn of humankind and that I really needed to acknowledge that primeval aspect, so making sounds really helped to get in touch with that.

Once the midwife had arrived and then left again, I felt better, and relieved that Hannah had been checked and that all was going to plan. Time was flying. It felt like the whole first stage was sort of a blur of sounds, movement, baths, hugs, homeopathy and, as the contractions grew stronger, the blessed TENS machine.

By about seven in the morning, the midwife was back, but Hannah still needed to dilate a little more and by nine o'clock she was ready to pass over to the morning shift midwives. I remember that I did my best to help keep Hannah focused on each contraction and not worry about the comings and goings of the people around us. At this stage I also became more aware of the environment as I could hear the neighbour's kids all leaving for school in between Hannah's screams. ('Maa' had turned to screams at some point – well, screaming 'Maa' anyway!)

By eleven o'clock, and into the second stage, Hannah was afraid the baby wasn't going to be able to make it out and kept on muttering, "It's impossible". What could I do but listen and support her on my shoulder. Mentally carrying on with mantras, I was praying that all would work out smoothly and that all the pain would be over soon!

We were beginning to have some encouraging signs as what seemed like the baby's head was beginning to show, but every time Hannah pushed, the baby couldn't seem to get past the point of no return. I kept on hoping that all would soon be over and that baby would arrive – though I could tell the contractions were getting further and further apart and also getting shorter. I was beginning to get worried, although of course didn't show any signs to Hannah, who was already in disbelief that the baby was going to make it.

As time went on the pattern continued: the baby's head beginning to show but not crowning. By 12:30 Jo, our midwife, told Hannah that she probably only had two contractions left and to make the most of them. It was at this point I knew that getting her to hospital right now was not going to be easy. So I mustered one final prayer, "Please help right now!" In one move, as Hannah turned round the baby's head appeared and the next moment he was in my hands. I passed him through Hannah's legs to her arms.

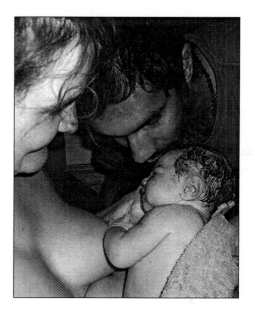

Here's when I remembered the second bit of advice given to me the week before: "Really feel that first touch." I'll never forget it. What a touch of beautiful Rohan, my son!

For another perspective on this experience, you can read Hannah's story on p.15

Chris's story

(a photo-essay)

Oliver, 1979

My wife, Corinne, and I started planning these photographs as soon as we had arranged for our fourth baby to be born at home. I had watched first Miranda and 16 months later our twins, Abigail and Verity, being born. Now I felt ready and able to photograph a birth.

Corinne was a teacher for the National Childbirth Trust. Her interest in the birth process, and enthusiasm for this project, made a vital contribution to the success of the photographs.

Oliver was born in our bedroom on the second floor of our house in Uxbridge.

It was a gloriously sunny Monday in March.

For another perspective on this experience, you can read Corinne's story on p.24

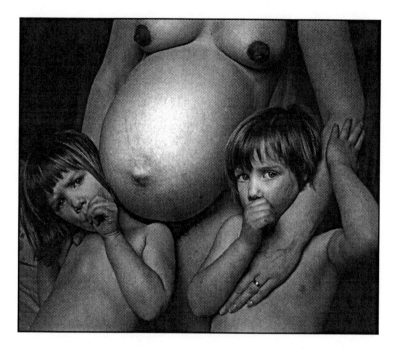

Sunday 11 March 1979

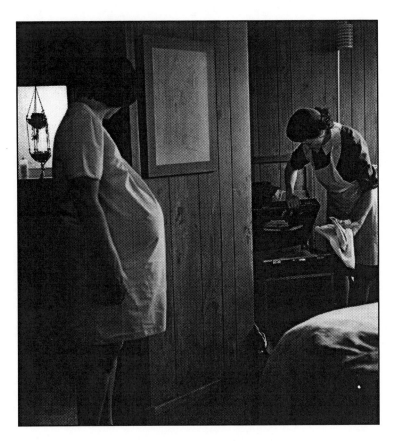

11:00am, Monday 12 March 1979

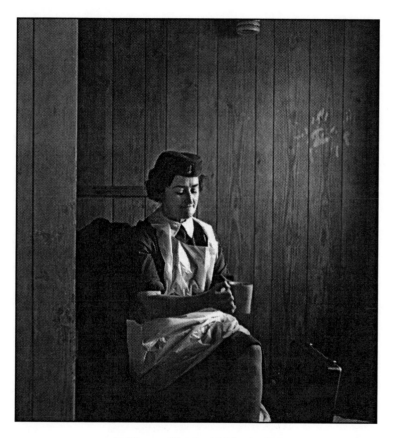

12:00 noon, Monday 12 March 1979

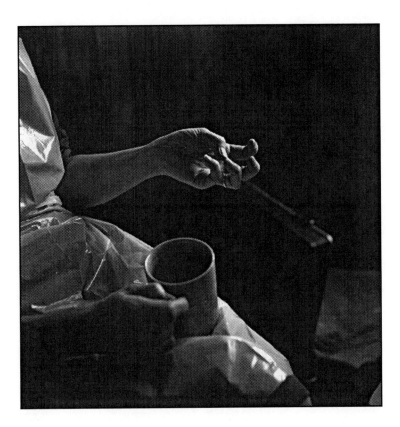

1:00pm, Monday 12 March 1979

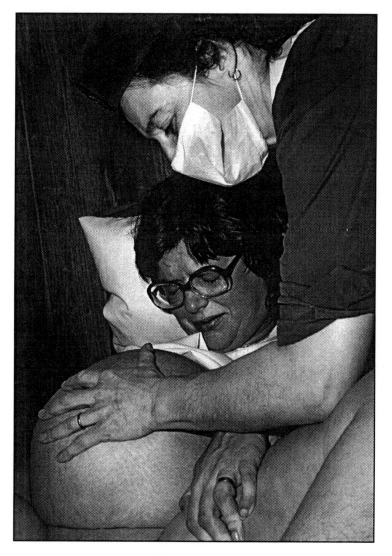

2:00pm, Monday 12 March 1979

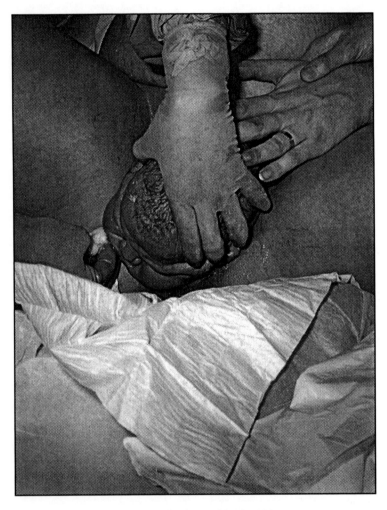

3:14pm, Monday 12 March 1979

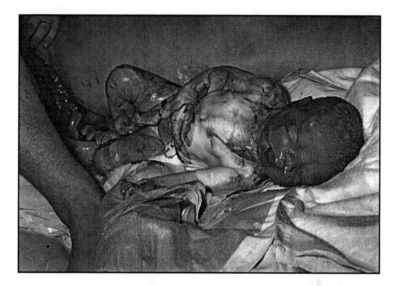

3:16pm, Monday 12 March 1979

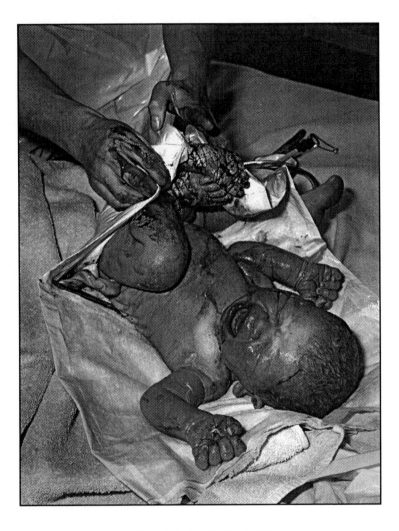

3:18pm, Monday 12 March 1979

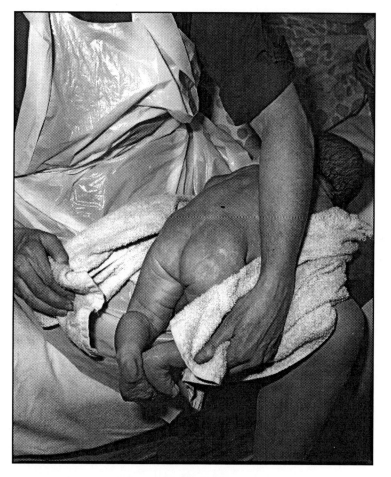

3:25pm, Monday 12 March 1979

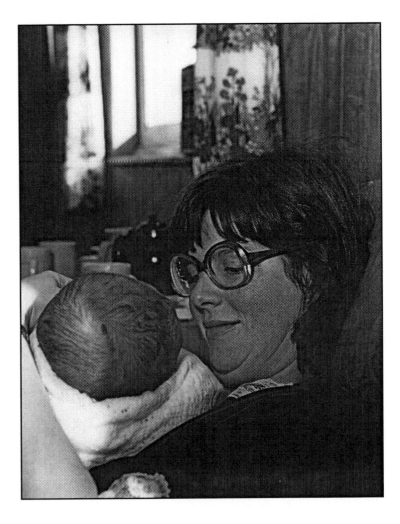

3:30pm, Monday 12 March 1979

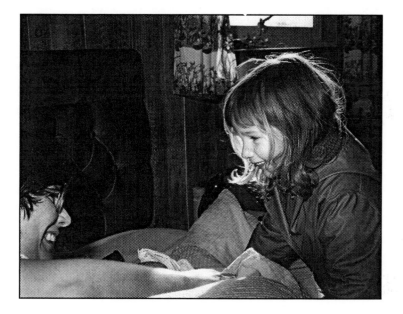

3:40pm, Monday 12 March 1979

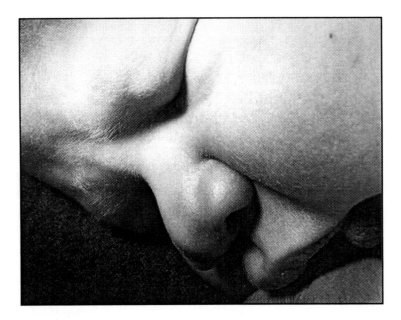

3:45pm, Monday 12 March 1979

Further reading

The list below includes books and websites that the contributors found especially useful.

Books

Active Birth
Janet Balaskas, Harvard Common Press, 1992

Am I Allowed?
Beverley Lawrence Beech, AIMS, 2003

Baby Catcher
Peggy Vincent, Simon & Schuster, 2003

Birth and Beyond
Dr Yehudi Gordon, Vermilion, 2002

Birth Reborn
Michel Odent, Souvenir Press, 1994

Birth Your Way
Sheila Kitzinger, Dorling Kindersley, 2002

Encyclopedia of Pregnancy and Birth
Janet Balaskas and Yehudi Gordon, Little, Brown, 1989

Hello Baby (A children's book about home birth)
Jenni Overend, Frances Lincoln, 2004

Ina May's Guide to Childbirth
Ina May Gaskin, Bantam USA, 2003

Preparing for Birth with Yoga
Janet Balaskas, HarperCollins, 2003

Rediscovering Birth
Sheila Kitzinger, Simon & Schuster, 2001

Spiritual Midwifery
Ina May Gaskin, Book Publishing Company, 2002

The Bloke's Guide to Pregnancy
Jon Smith, Hay House, 2004

Websites

Active Birth Centre
Provides information on pregnancy, active, home and water birth, breastfeeding, mother and babycare.
www.activebirthcentre.com

Association for Improvements in the Maternity Services
Campaigns for normal birth and provides information about maternity choices in the UK and Ireland.
www.aims.org.uk

Association of Radical Midwives
A support group for UK midwives who are committed to improving maternity care within the NHS, and for women who cannot find the care they need.
www.radmid.demon.co.uk

Baby Centre
A UK resource for pregnancy and parenting, including a home birth forum.
www.babycentre.co.uk

Baby Whisperer International
A portal to help support parents and families.
www.babywhisperer.com

Birth Choice UK
Gives maternity statistics for NHS hospitals in the UK.
www.birthchoiceuk.com

Birth-Pool-in-a-Box
Aims to increase access to water birth at home by making birth pools more affordable.
www.birthpoolinabox.co.uk

Bump to Baby
Provider of birth and parenting courses for individual couples.
www.bumptobaby.org

Doula UK
Information about lay birth partners and how to find a doula.
www.doula.org.uk

The Good Birth Company
Supplier of active birth equipment and feeding accessories.
www.thegoodbirth.co.uk

Home Birth Reference Site
Provides information about home birth for parents and health professionals
www.homebirth.org.uk

Independent Midwives Association
Website includes facility to find a midwife and provides clinical statistics.
www.independentmidwives.org.uk

La Leche League
An international breastfeeding support group.
www.laleche.org.uk

Natal Hypnotherapy
A resource for courses and hypnotherapy CDs.
www.natalhypnotherapy.co.uk

National Childbirth Trust
Organisation promoting normal birth and providing antenatal classes, breastfeeding support and an online shop.
www.nct.org.uk

UK Parents
A pregnancy and parenting resource which includes a home birth forum.
www.ukparents.co.uk

Yoga Birth
Yoga and antenatal classes for pregnancy.
yogabirth.co.uk

Author credits

Thanks to: Rachel Ainley-Carruthers; Abigail Cairns; Tom Cairns; Joyce Collings; Phill Collings; Sarah Collings; Mark Cousins; Pamela Davis; Andy Derrick; Mary Derrick; Tracii Edwards; Sarah Ellis; Deborah Faulkner; Hannah Fries; Chris Holmes; Corinne Holmes; Pam Holmes; Victoria Hood; Laura Jones; Lucy Joyce; Sue Lawther; Andrea Lee; Hannah Luck; Ameet Malhotra; Sarah Osborn; Carla Page; Sarah Salzano; Hannah Sawtell; Melissa Scott; Paul Taylor; Tracy Taylor; Ann Waite; Julie Walford; Nicki Wilkinson; and to those who chose to remain anonymous.